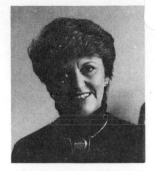

Ann Watson, M Inst H Ec, taught cookery in the Department of Community Education at Tile Hill College of Further Education, Coventry, where she ran popular international and wholefood cookery courses as well as teaching disabled people to cook following the recommended healthy eating guidelines. She now works full-time as a freelance cookery writer and home economist and is local tutor for the British Diabetic Association, for whom she holds diabetic cookery classes. She is married and has three children.

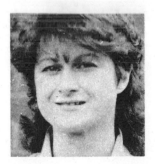

Sue Lousley, BSc, SRD, was Research Nutritionist and Chief Dietitian at the Radcliffe Infirmary, Oxford. She worked with Dr Jim Mann in his diabetic unit, where the high-fibre, low-fat diabetic diet was first introduced in the UK. She is coauthor of *Diabetic Delights*. Now a Nutrition Consultant, she is married and has one child.

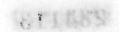

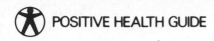 POSITIVE HEALTH GUIDE

THE DIABETICS' INTERNATIONAL DIET BOOK

Ann Watson and Sue Lousley

Foreword by
Dr Jim Mann, DM, PhD
Honorary Consultant Physician
The John Radcliffe Hospital, Oxford

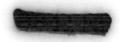

O P T I M A

First published in 1987 by Macdonald Optima
a division of Macdonald & Co. (Publishers) Ltd

British Library Cataloguing in Publication Data

Watson, Ann.
   The diabetics' international diet book.
   – (Positive health guide)
   I. Diabetes – Diet therapy – Recipes.
   I. Title. II. Lousley, Sue. III. Series
   651.5'6314   RC662

ISBN 0 356 14739 8

Macdonald & Co. (Publishers) Ltd
3rd Floor
Greater London House
Hampstead Road
London NW1 7QX

A BPLC PLC Company

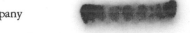

Acknowledgements are due to Ray Moller for the photography, assisted by Sophie
Butt; Valerie Wright for art direction; Sue Russell for styling; and Lisa Collard for
food preparation.

Front cover photograph shows: Tim suen yeh choi sa lud (top left, see page 105);
Salsa guacamole (top right, see page 49); Murgh tandoori (see page 70).

Back cover photograph shows: Kenchin jiru (see page 31).

Printed by Toppan Printing Company (S) Pte Ltd, Singapore

CONTENTS

FOREWORD

Dr Jim Mann, DM PhD
Honorary Consultant Physician
The John Radcliffe Hospital, Oxford

The idea of a high-fibre low-fat diet for diabetics was first introduced in the mid 1970s. Changing from the old-fashioned low-carbohydrate diet to this way of eating resulted in improved blood sugar levels and lower levels of blood cholesterol. At first the idea of a high-carbohydrate diet for people with diabetes was regarded as heretical, but now high-fibre low-fat diets are recommended by National Diabetes Associations throughout the world.

Several books in the Positive Health Guide series have played a major role in showing that this way of eating can be enjoyable as well as healthy, but *The Diabetics' International Diet Book* breaks new ground. There is increasing interest in recipes from other countries but unfortunately many are high in fat and highly processed carbohydrate. They are therefore not suitable for people with diabetes or, indeed, others wishing to follow a healthy way of eating. This book starts with a fascinating introduction which describes eating habits and favourite recipes around the world. It explains how they can be adapted for healthy eating while retaining the authentic flavours. There follows a collection of recipes from Latin America, the Middle and Far East which will satisfy those who already have adventurous tastes and will offer an irresistible opportunity for experimentation to those who have not yet done so.

This book is a must for diabetics, their families and any others who wish to eat well and stay healthy.

INTRODUCTION

Eating is now a far more elaborate business than ever before. Gone are the days of the standard meat and two vegetables – roast meat on Sunday, cold meat on Monday and fish on Friday. People are becoming more adventurous and enthusiastic about what they eat, a change in attitudes reflected in the number and variety of restaurants which have sprung up, particularly in large cities. The traditional styles of cooking – English, French, Italian – remain popular but there is increasing experimentation with more exotic foods. Chinese and Indian restaurants are now commonplace and there is a growing number of Middle Eastern restaurants, especially Greek and Turkish, while many highly specialized restaurants, such as Iranian, Egyptian, Indonesian and Thai, have started to appear. Similarly, previously unknown foods are available in outlets ranging from delicatessens and health food stores to ethnic market stalls and corner shops. Even general supermarkets now stock dried beans, pitta bread and spices, which ten or fifteen years ago were unknown outside their country of origin.

Trying new restaurants and new styles of cooking is fun and straightforward for the majority: the only relevant question is whether you like it or not. However, for those on a special diet, eating new and unknown dishes can cause problems. What are the ingredients and are they suitable? Of course, unless you are allergic to a specific food, it does not matter if you occasionally eat something that is not considered advisable on your diet, although being unsure about what you are eating can spoil your enjoyment. This is not confined to eating out. Many people who would otherwise like to try cooking new dishes are reluctant to do so because of the restrictions of specialized diets, whether they be weight-reducing, diabetic or cholesterol-lowering. If you are on a calorie- or carbohydrate-controlled diet it is certainly not easy to calculate the nutritional content of more complicated meals, so for many people with diabetes it is often simpler, if less enjoyable, to stick to the old tried and tested recipes.

The aim of this book is to change all that. We have explained in previous publications how a low-fat, high-fibre diet can be interesting and appetizing and how cakes and biscuits can be included in the diabetic diet (*The Diabetics' Diet Book*, *The Diabetics' Cookbook*, and *Diabetic Delights*, also in this series). Now we would like to show you how you can enjoy an international cuisine that is delicious, wholesome and different.

WHAT IS DIABETES?

There are several forms of diabetes but they are all caused by a lack of effective insulin, a hormone produced by the pancreas. Insulin has a number of functions, one of which is to enable sugar to be removed from the bloodstream to the tissues, where it is used to supply energy. Lack of insulin leads to high levels of sugar in the bloodstream – known as hyperglycaemia – and to other changes in the body's metabolism.

There are two main forms of diabetes, of which the most common is non-insulin dependent diabetes mellitus (NIDDM) or maturity-onset diabetes. This condition almost always develops in middle age and is usually associated with at least some degree of overweight, and frequently serious obesity. People with this type of diabetes are able to produce some insulin but it cannot be used effectively. This less severe form of the condition can be controlled by diet alone or by diet combined with oral hypoglycaemic agents (tablets), so injections of insulin are rarely required.

A less common condition is insulin-dependent diabetes mellitus (IDDM) or juvenile-onset diabetes. This usually develops in children and young people, when the pancreas completely loses its ability to produce insulin. The symptoms tend to develop much more quickly than in NIDDM and to be more severe. People with IDDM have to take daily insulin injections but for them too diet has an important role to play.

THE DIABETES–DIET CONNECTION

The overwhelming diet-related factor in the development of NIDDM appears to be obesity. The high fat (and therefore calorie) content of the foods consumed in Westernized countries is in striking contrast to the diets of people living in traditional agricultural or subsistence societies. This is partly due to the popularity of processed and convenience products with a high fat content and little or no fibre: the lack of fibre means that, to satisfy the appetite, large quantities of this high-calorie food need to be consumed. The resulting high total calorie intake is thought to lead to obesity, which is very strongly associated with NIDDM: this is the suggested link between high energy intake and diabetes.

People who have already developed diabetes also need to watch their weight for a number of important reasons:

- For people with NIDDM, losing weight seems partially to overcome insulin resistance and so is very important in controlling their condition. Injected insulin works more efficiently when people with IDDM are not overweight.
- Maintaining normal weight reduces the risk of heart disease, which is more common among people with either type of diabetes than among nondiabetics.

Other dietary factors apart from total energy intake have been associated with the development of diabetes. Of these, a high refined sucrose intake and low intake of dietary fibre are probably of most significance – but there is still a great deal of controversy.

There is no doubt, however, that all these dietary factors play a very important part in the treatment of both types of diabetes once they have developed.

A HEALTHY DIET FOR DIABETICS – AND THE WHOLE FAMILY

In recent years, the frightening increase in 'diseases of affluence' (such as heart disease, certain cancers and diabetes) in Westernized countries has forced a reassessment of our eating habits and led to attempts to improve our diet. It is now obvious that we eat too much fat, sugar and salt and too little unrefined carbohydrate: recently developed health guidelines in both the UK and the USA reflect this view, and aim to reverse the trend.

These dietary goals, though directed at the whole population, are in fact very similar to those that have been recommended by doctors and dietitians for people with diabetes since the late 1970s, with the only real difference being the greater emphasis for diabetics on sugar restriction. The modern diabetic diet (described in *The Diabetics' Diet Book* – also in this series) emphasizes a high-carbohydrate-and-fibre but low fat approach. One of its most important features is that it not only helps to control blood sugar levels but is also generally good for health and therefore recommended for the whole family.

The new direction

A carbohydrate-restricted diet has been traditionally recommended for diabetics but recent research has shown that it is not actually necessary. A diet high in starchy (but not sugary) carbohydrate can in fact improve blood sugar levels and reduce the risk of diabetes and its complications. Cereals, vegetables and fruits provide most of the carbohydrate, and these also contain substantial quantities of dietary fibre. It is now accepted that a generous dietary fibre intake protects against constipation and many bowel diseases. Even more important for diabetics is that sugar absorption is further slowed by dietary fibre, so a combination of high-starch and high-fibre foods (especially those like the various dried beans, containing leguminous fibre) offers the best chance for dietary control. As a bonus, this type of diet aids weight control by making it easier to reduce the amount of fat consumed (especially saturated animal fat).

Apart from sugar, or sucrose, which in its refined form should be avoided on the diabetic diet, fat is the constituent that should be most severely restricted. Since this plays a part in the international cuisines in this book, we should look at fats more closely.

WHAT IS FAT?

The term can cause confusion because it covers a variety of substances including solid visible fats such as butter, lard and margarine; the invisible fats in red meat, cheese, milk and oils, both vegetable and fish. It also includes fat in the body, where it is the fuel store and also part of the essential structure of cells. In the body there are two main forms of fat.

Cholesterol

This is not a true fat as it does not contain fatty acids. It is a waxy, fat-like substance which is produced mainly in the liver. It is transported by the bloodstream to cells throughout the body where it is essential for the production of hormones, vitamin D, cell membranes and the sheaths that protect nerve fibres. The liver itself needs cholesterol to make bile acids which help in the digestion of fats. Although cholesterol is an essential part of the body's make up, it is not an essential part of the diet. The body can produce all the cholesterol it needs from the food we eat without eating cholesterol itself. The danger is in fact that too much cholesterol is produced by the body. This causes raised levels in the blood (hypercholesterolaemia) which can lead to deposits of cholesterol in the artery walls. If this happens to the main arteries supplying the heart, and narrowing of these arteries occurs, a heart attack can result. There is a definite association between high blood cholesterol levels and coronary heart disease. When this association first became evident it was automatically assumed that cholesterol in the food made the biggest contribution to cholesterol levels in the blood. Since then it has become apparent that this makes up only a very small part of the total blood cholesterol. The concentration of cholesterol is affected much more by the amount and type of true fat that we eat.

Triglycerides

The main form in which fats occur both in food and in the body is as complex molecules called triglycerides. These are made up of three smaller molecules called fatty acids which are responsible for the different physical natures of the fats and oils.

What are fatty acids?   Fatty acids are made up of carbon, hydrogen and oxygen atoms. Each carbon atom has four bonds with which it can attach atoms of hydrogen. If all four bonds are attached to hydrogen atoms, the fatty acid is said to be *saturated* as no further bonding with hydrogen can occur. If bonds are available to attach to more hydrogen atoms the fatty acid is *monounsaturated*. *Polyunsaturated* fatty acids are those that can attach four or more additional hydrogen atoms. Therefore these have two or more double bonds in their molecular structure, compared with the one double bond of monounsaturated fatty acids. When saturated, no double bonds exist. The diagram below shows how the different fatty acids are formed.

It is the degree of unsaturation of the fatty acids that plays an important part in determining the physical nature of the fat. Fats consisting mainly of saturated fatty acids are solid at room temperature, while those with a high proportion of unsaturated fats are usually liquid. No fat is made up entirely of one type of fatty acid. However, animal fats generally contain a high proportion of saturated fatty acids, while vegetable and fish oils tend to have a high monounsaturated and polyunsaturated content. Corn oil, sunflower oil, safflower oil and soya oil are particularly high in polyunsaturated fatty acids and nuts and olives have a predominantly monounsaturated content. There are of course exceptions to this rule. For example, coconut and palm oils both have a high saturated fatty acid content.

Fatty acids and health   It is now well established that saturated fatty acids increase blood cholesterol levels while polyunsaturated fatty acids tend to reduce them. It is generally accepted that monounsaturated fats do not affect blood cholesterol levels one way or the other. As already mentioned, high blood cholesterol levels are strongly associated with a greater risk of coronary heart disease. As more research is done, however, the picture becomes more complicated. One example is the question of the role of monounsaturated fatty acids. Some studies suggest that populations consuming large quantities of olive oil, with its high monounsaturated fatty acid content, have a low incidence of heart disease and that monounsaturated fats lower blood cholesterol levels. Although much has been made of this recently in the popular press, the evidence is certainly not conclusive and it is still generally thought that monounsaturated fats remain 'in the middle'.

Studies of the polyunsaturated fats have also become more involved. Over the last twenty-five years or so the fatty acid most strongly associated with low blood cholesterol levels has been linoleic acid. This is found in large quantities in corn, soya, sunflower seed and safflower seed oils. It is made by plants but not by animals. Recommendations for lowering blood cholesterol levels have concentrated on increasing the proportion of this fatty acid in the diet.

Recently, however, interest has increased in a polyunsaturated fatty acid called eicosapentaenoic acid — EPA for short. Fish oils contain large amounts of EPA and populations that eat large amounts of fish or marine mammals, such as Greenland Eskimos, the Japanese and coastal Turks, have a high intake of EPA. These populations have significantly lower rates of coronary heart disease than Western populations. In Japan where the death rates from coronary heart disease are low, the lowest rates are found on the island of Okinawa where fish consumption is about twice as high as on the mainland of Japan (where the average intake is 100g fish per person per day). Studies have shown that these fish-eating populations have lower levels of blood triglycerides and higher levels of high density lipoprotein or HDL compared with populations that eat only small amounts of fish. HDL is thought to protect against coronary heart disease by removing unnecessary cholesterol from the bloodstream and preventing it from being deposited on the artery walls, so reducing the risk of narrowed arteries.

All these changes in blood 'fats' have been associated with a reduced risk of coronary heart disease. These points are important for everyone but they are particularly relevant to people with diabetes who are especially at risk from coronary heart disease.

FAR EASTERN, MIDDLE EASTERN AND LATIN AMERICAN CUISINE

There is a marked contrast in the prevalence of diabetes between the Westernized and the developing world (2 to 4 per cent against 1 to 2 per cent). Although genetic factors are thought to play a part in explaining this difference, diabetes, as a disease of affluence, accurately reflects a society's lifestyle.

Generally speaking, the more developed a society, the more likely is the population to eat an undesirably high-energy, low-fibre diet. The table opposite compares the nutrients available for consumption in the UK and the USA with those in some of the countries whose recipes are used in this book. Although separate fibre figures are not available, an idea can be gained by comparing the carbohydrate and fat intakes. Fibre is provided only by plant foods – cereals, vegetables and fruits – which are high in carbohydrate and low in fat, so as a rule, the higher the carbohydrate content of the diet, the greater the dietary fibre intake.

In countries such as Greece, Japan, China, India and the Middle East, people eat more vegetables, fruit, cereals and fish and a lot less meat and fat. Oil, and less of it, is used rather than hard fats in cooking. The average Japanese or Mexican obtains less than one-third of his daily calories from fat and of this a high proportion is of vegetable or fish origin. This compares with over 40 per cent of calories coming from fat in the UK or US diet, much of which is of animal origin. It is hardly surprising that affluence-related diseases take such a toll.

The use of processed and convenience foods sets apart the eating habits of Westerners from those of more rural societies. The diets of many of the countries included here are necessarily determined by what foods are produced on the land rather than by what is manufactured or imported and the majority of these cuisines have remained virtually unchanged over many hundreds of years. There are many similarities in the cooking methods of the different nations and also many fascinating variations. To understand and enjoy the recipes it is important to know at least something of the culinary traditions of these countries.

China

Chinese cooking is probably the best known of the Asian cuisines. However, traditional Chinese cooking is far more precise and exacting than is often exhibited in the average suburban Chinese restaurant. In China, cooking and eating are taken very seriously: good cooks are highly regarded and cooking is considered an art. There is not one cuisine, but several regional varieties, which is not surprising in such a vast country with extremes of geography and climate. In addition, the variety of races inhabiting China over centuries has resulted in many different styles of cooking.

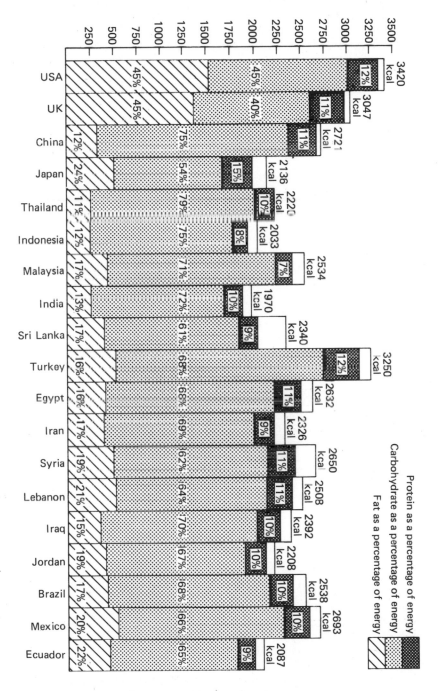

Comparison of nutrients available per person per day

The basic difference is between the north and south: a major agricultural division exists. In the north wheat and other grain products are eaten, while in the south rice is the staple food. More precise differences have arisen between north, south, east and west and, gradually, five different styles of cooking have evolved.

Peking or Shantung style (northern)   The emphasis is on delicate flavours and the food is light and mildly seasoned. Since wheat, millet and barley are the staple crops, noodles, dumplings and steamed buns are the main source of carbohydrate. It is from this style of cooking that the famous Peking Duck and also spring rolls originated.

Honan style (northern)   Honan province is famous for its sweet and sour dishes and also for its Yellow River Carp. Unlike Peking-style cooking, the food is highly spiced.

Cantonese style (southern)   Kwantung is the southern province of China, with a tropical climate and the longest sea coast of all the provinces. Canton, a centre for foreign trade, has produced some of the best-known Chinese dishes. A characteristic feature of this cooking is that the main component of a dish is frequently cooked whole rather than diced. It is here that the more exotic dishes, using shark fins, lobsters and birds' nests, originated. Vegetable rather than meat dishes are popular and stir-frying is the most common method of cooking.

Fukien style (eastern)   The best-known dishes from this area are the 'red cooked' foods: the ingredients are simmered slowly in soy sauce until the liquid evaporates, leaving a reddish tinge to the food. Some of the wonderful clear soups and sweet and sour dishes have their origins here. With a subtropical climate, the staple food is rice, although in the northern area around Shanghai, wheat and barley are grown. Preserved foods such as fish, mushrooms and the famous 'hundred-year-old' buried eggs are said to have originated here.

Szechwan style (western)   Western China's cuisine is characterized by hot and spicy flavours and shows many similarities to the food of Thailand and Burma. The area is fertile and is known as 'the land of abundance'. A large variety of vegetables and cereals is grown and game and freshwater fish are common.

Although the styles of cooking may differ between regions, the theme of economy is common throughout China. The basis of traditional Chinese cooking has been to conserve fuel, to make a little food go a long way and to use everything that is edible to good effect. China's land area is similar to that of the USA but only 12 per cent is arable. Added to this is China's huge population which puts a considerable strain on food resources. In order to feed everybody the Chinese have learned to make the maximum possible use of everything available.

To get the most out of the precious fuel, two styles of cooking have evolved. Chao or stir-frying is the stirring and tossing of small pieces of food over a fierce heat. A wok is used which, with its convex shape, makes it easy to toss the ingredients and also enables the use of small quantities of oil. Since a large surface area is exposed to direct heat and the food is cut into small pieces, cooking time is short and little fuel is used. This does mean, however, that all the food must be prepared prior to cooking. Success depends on the careful chopping of the food so that it is all of a similar size, and on the sequence of adding ingredients, so that foods such as meat, which take longer to cook, are added first. This type of cooking cannot be done in advance as, if the food is left warming, it will continue to cook in its own heat. Stir-fried vegetables should be crisp, and good quality meat and fish should be just cooked and juicy. In contrast, slow-simmering is used to tenderize tough, inferior cuts of meat, stewing them in liquid for several hours together with root vegetables. This method traditionally uses the dying embers of the fire and thus again conserves fuel.

Economy in the use of ingredients is achieved by eating everything edible: a feature of Chinese cuisine is the variety of ingredients used, from dried wood fungus, lily buds and lotus seeds, to birds' nests in soups. (The nests are not in fact made from twigs, but from the saliva of a small type of swift; the nests have to be gathered from highly inaccessible cliffs and require a great deal of preparation. As a result, birds' nest soup is an expensive delicacy and is only served at banquets and on special occasions.)

One other important point affecting the Chinese diet is their ancient association of food and health. Healthy eating is a relatively new idea in the West but an old Chinese proverb runs, 'He that takes medicine and neglects diet wastes the skill of the physician'. The ancient Chinese linked the five flavours of food – sweet, sour, bitter, hot and salty – with the five basic elements – earth, wood, fire, metal and water. These were referred back to the human body by identifying them with the stomach, liver, heart, lungs and kidneys. It was believed that food has different, specific effects on health in addition to providing nourishment. Health is affected if the harmony of the body is upset by the introduction of the wrong foods. Some foods were considered opposed or incompatible with each other and balance was important. Yin, meaning cool, shaded, the weaker force, should be balanced with Yang, all that is strong and hot. Food was characterized as either Yin or Yang and, when the two are in balance, harmony and tranquillity are achieved, and consequently good health. Too much of one causes imbalance and ill health. Furthermore, specific foods such as garlic and ginseng were thought to be of particular benefit.

These venerable Chinese traditions now form the basis of healthy eating for many people around the world. The exact pattern may not be followed (as in, for example, Britain's healthy eating guidelines), but the general principles are the same. Over-indulgence of any food can be harmful and a balance of nutrients is necessary for good health.

Japan

Japanese food is unique and stands apart from all other Asian cooking. It has retained completely its traditional and ethnic style of cooking, uninfluenced by other countries. The Japanese as a nation remained almost totally isolated from the rest of the world until the middle of the last century, unlike Asian nations of the mainland whose cultures and cuisines became intermingled with those of their neighbours. This isolation perpetuated a simple cuisine, relying on the indigenous foods of the country, that has remained virtually unchanged through the centuries. Since little land is available for agriculture, the Japanese have come to treat their food with care and to appreciate quality over quantity. Meals are served in small portions and are always beautifully presented. Often a theme is adopted for a meal and the table and food will be decorated and garnished accordingly, using such adornments as radish flowers, a spray of pine needles or perhaps a single chrysanthemum flower or leaf. The visual aspect, with its interplay of colours, shapes and textures, is as important as the flavour of the foods.

The isolation of the Japanese and the restrictions of the limited agricultural land have also been responsible for the greatest difference between Japanese and other Asian cuisines. With a comparatively limited variety of foodstuffs available, a culinary tradition has developed that emphasizes the flavour of the individual foods and variety in the method of preparation. Unlike the Chinese and other Asians, who blend herbs and spices with the main ingredients to give a bouquet of flavours, the Japanese prefer to maintain the purity of each ingredient. Because of this, it is very important that the food is completely fresh and the Japanese tend to shop every day to ensure this.

Another difference is that much of Japanese cooking is done over water with far less use of oil and fat than in other cuisines. This is thought to be one of the reasons why the Japanese, as a race, are slim and healthy with a low incidence of heart disease; although the saltiness of their food has been linked with another common condition, stroke. The Japanese recipes in this book keep the addition of salt to the minimum, following the recommended guidelines for healthy eating.

Since food is rarely roasted or baked and most cooking is done on top of the stove, timing is essential. As in Chinese cooking, ingredients are cut into small pieces and then steamed, boiled, fried or grilled. Similarly, the food has to be cooked immediately before serving and should not be kept warming. As with most Asian meals, the Japanese do not serve their food in courses but set all the dishes out at the start of the meal.

Traditionally, the diet of the Japanese has been simple and based on fish, vegetables, rice, fruit and seaweed, though meat was included from time to time, when available. On the few occasions when the Japanese made contact with other races, new foods were introduced to the country, such as soybeans and tea from China. In the 1850s the Japanese were forced to forego their insular attitude and with a broader outlook came some changes in their cuisine. The Shinto tenets of vegetarianism were gradually abandoned and beef, pork and poultry began to be used more regularly. However fish, soybean products, seaweed, vegetables, rice and fruit remain the basis of Japanese cuisine.

Fish and seafood are eaten at every meal; they are always fresh and no meal is complete without them. Raw fish is very popular and, although this may not sound very appetizing, its freshness and quality ensures that there is no hint of 'fishiness' in either odour or flavour. Sushi and sashini are the two styles of serving uncooked fish. Sushi is fish in lightly vinegared rice, garnished with either raw or cooked fish and seafood, strips of seaweed, vegetables and egg. Sashini consists of cuts of the finest fish, garnished with crisp shavings of daikon (a long white radish) and dipped into soy sauce and wasabi (a hot, green, creamy horseradish). There is a vast variety of fish available in Japan, including tuna, mackerel, salmon, halibut, sea bass, porgy, red snapper, eel, squid, octopus and clams.

The three main soybean products – miso, tofu and shoyu – are another major source of protein in the Japanese diet. Miso is a savoury paste made from fermented soy beans. Tofu or bean curd is made from soybean milk and is often used to garnish soups. Shoyu (soy sauce), an extract of soy beans, wheat, barley, salt, malt and water, is used to flavour Japanese food as well as the foods of most other Asian countries.

Seaweed is a popular and tasty Japanese food which is normally eaten wrapped around fish and other foods, or as a garnish in a variety of snacks, including rice crackers. The two principal seaweeds are nori (laver) and kombi (kelp), a vital ingredient in the Japanese stock called dashi. The main carbohydrate in the Japanese diet is rice, but udon (wheat noodles) and soba (buckwheat noodles) are also used.

Thailand

The staple crop in Thailand is rice but coconut is also very important and coconut milk* forms part of almost all Thai dishes, from curries to desserts and beverages. The main source of protein is fish which is eaten both fresh and dried, in which form it can be kept for a considerable time without refrigeration.

In their cooking style, as well as in their religion and culture, the Thai people have absorbed many foreign ideas: Thai cuisine blends Chinese, Indian, and Arabic influences. The dominant method of cooking is stir-frying with a wok and, as with the Chinese, the balance of the five flavours – sweet, sour, bitter, hot and salty – is very important. A typical Thai meal consists of an assortment of curry dishes, soups, salads, vegetables and sauces, served simultaneously around a central bowl of boiled rice. Desserts are generally reserved for formal dinners and normally fruit is served at the end of the meal.

Indonesia

The cuisine of Indonesia has been strongly influenced by India, by Arab traders, the Chinese and the Dutch as a result of strong links with the spice trade. Indonesia is the world's largest island chain, comprising nearly 13,700 islands, of which Sumatra, Java, Kalimantan and Celebes are the

*Coconut milk is the liquid expressed from the flesh of the coconut after it has been soaked in boiling water or milk. It is not the liquid found in fresh coconut.

largest. Unlike China and other Asian countries, there is no real *haute cuisine* and most of the dishes have originated from the peasantry. Rice is eaten at every meal and is the staple food, supplemented by corn, sago, sweet potatoes and coconuts. The cooking style varies from region to region and island to island. Sumatra has been influenced by Indian and Arab cuisine and its meals are more substantial, with pilau type rices, meat curries and very spicy food. Javan food is more subtle, often with combinations of sweet, sour and hot flavours. The Javans have a sweet tooth and eat a lot of cakes, sweets and sweetmeats. The cuisine of the smaller islands has been influenced more by Malaysia and Polynesia and tends to be less exotic.

Feasts are a common feature of Indonesian life. In the past the focal point of the feast was often a huge dish of festival rice, tinted yellow with turmeric. The rijstaffel (or rice table) originated with the opulent banquets given by the Dutch, where sixty or seventy dishes were served around the central rice dish. However, with independence the rijstaffel became unpopular with the Indonesian natives because of its association with foreign domination. It is still served in some restaurants and at buffets in luxury hotels, but it is aimed at the tourist trade and is no longer a part of Indonesian culture.

As in many other Asian countries, to the Indonesians, colour, texture and flavour are all equally important. Meals are carefully balanced and spicy foods are offset by bland ones, soft foods by crisp and wet by dry.

Indian

Indian cooking style and eating patterns have largely been dictated by geography, climate and religious influences. The main agricultural split, and therefore the most marked division in Indian cuisine, is between the north and south. The staple food in the north is wheat, which is used mainly for the Indian breads such as chapati, poori, naan and paratha. The northern cuisine has been influenced by that of Iran, resulting in a combination of Hindu and Muslim styles, while the southern diet is rice-based. Meat is excluded from the diet of high-caste Hindus, and Buddhists, who believe in reincarnation; and pork and shellfish from the diet of Muslims. Because of these taboos, vegetables play a very important part in Indian cuisine so that many main dishes are ideally suited to the diabetic diet. Indian vegetarian dishes, such as the bhaji (fried vegetables), bartha (purées) and pakoras (fritters), are in a class of their own.

Not even vegetables are exempt from dietary taboos among some Indian people. Garlic, considered so beneficial to the health in China, is forbidden in some parts of India as, along with onions, it 'inflames the passions and heats the blood'. Tomatoes and beetroot are not eaten by some because of their bloodlike colour.

Curries   The oustanding feature of all Indian cooking is the use of highly flavoured spices throughout the subcontinent. Certainly, to most people Indian cooking means curries. Curries are merely dishes made aromatic with spices and then simmered slowly or stewed over a low heat with a lot of liquid. They can be hot or mild, subtle or pungent. Kormas, often described as dry curries, use only a small amount of stock, yoghurt or cream which is absorbed into the vegetables or meat. Indians tend to serve curries as everyday meals and use kormas for entertaining.

Tandoori Tandoori dishes, originating from the Punjab, are roasted or baked. A tandoor is a clay oven, which traditionally is sunk up to the neck in the ground. Nowadays it is often covered in a thick layer of plaster instead for extra insulation. Burning charcoal is placed in the bottom of the tandoor and the food, marinaded in spices, is speared on long spits. The best substitute for a tandoor oven is a charcoal barbecue or, failing that, a grill can be used.

Other cooking techniques Both shallow frying (bhoona) and deep frying (talawa) are used in Indian cooking. Steaming (dum) is often used in conjunction with other cooking methods. For example, the ingredients may be sautéed lightly with spices in a wok and then transferred with some liquid to a casserole and dummed for several hours or even overnight, over a dying stove. The traditional Indian stove, or chula, does not have an oven and so food is cooked on top with burning coals heaped on specially shaped lids for stewing and steaming.

Many of the Indian dishes which are fried tend to be too high in fat for people with diabetes, and so the recipes for them in this book have been specially converted. Thus you can eat these delicious Indian delicacies without upsetting your diet.

Cereals There are numerous rice dishes, such as pilau rice (originally from Persia) and biryanis in which rice is cooked with spices and vegetables or meat. Kitchri is a combination of rice, lentils and sometimes vegetables. Where rice is the staple food, it is always served in the centre of the plate and the curries and other accompaniments are placed around it. The proportion of rice to curries is important. Unlike in Western meals, where there tend to be large amounts of meat or fish and a small amount of rice, for Indians it is the other way around. Rice is the base and the curries should be served in much smaller portions. This is not only healthier but the highly spiced food needs the bland rice to balance it. Where wheat is the main cereal grown, Indian unleavened breads such as chapati, naan and paratha are served. The meal is eaten with the fingers, using the bread as a scoop for the accompaniments.

The main meal in India is eaten at midday; only banquets and very special meals are eaten at night. All the dishes are served at once except at banquets where the food is served in courses. The meal is accompanied by chatni (chutney) and raita (fresh vegetables or fruit in yoghurt). The only category of food eaten outside the home is snacks. These include samosa (fine pastry turnovers filled with spiced vegetables or meat), wada (deep fried crisp balls of lentils, onions and spices) and sev (deep fried crunchy noodles spiced with tumeric and cayenne pepper). There are hundreds of savoury snacks and sweetmeats. One thing Indian snacks have in common with our snacks, however, is that they invariably have a very high fat content. Mostly they are not suitable for the diabetic diet.

Middle East

The Middle East comprises a number of countries differing geographically and culturally. The lifestyles of the peoples vary from the completely Westernized to the traditional, subsistence existence of the Bedouin tribes, unchanged for centuries. The most Westernized areas are Israel, the Lebanon and the Caucasus but about 80 per cent of Middle Eastern people are peasants and of these a number are nomads. There are three main religions: Judaism, Christianity and Islam. Islam, which predominates, has a fundamental influence on daily life. Because of the dietary laws, pork and alcohol are not consumed by the majority of Middle Eastern people.

The cuisines of the countries throughout the Middle East have a great deal in common and often the differences tend to be between town and country rather than across borders because of the countries' shared history. Four main cooking styles have evolved of which the Iranian cuisine is the most refined and is the source of much of the *haute cuisine* of the Middle East. It is based on the long grain rice which grows around the Caspian Sea. The cuisines of Syria, Jordan and the Lebanon are similar. Turkish cooking is the one which has influenced most Westernized countries and has been known the longest. The fourth distinctive style of cooking is the Moroccan cuisine from North Africa where couscous (a type of granulated wheat) is the staple cereal.

Utensils and the type of heat available have determined the cuisine to a large extent. Ovens have only recently been introduced into most homes. In the past, cooking was done over a primitive stove called a fatayel. This was a long, slow procedure and food was often left to simmer overnight. It was often the practice in the past to send some dishes to be cooked in the large ovens of the local bakery and this still happens occasionally today, but for the most part dishes such as roast lamb, surrounded by vegetables, are cooked very slowly in domestic ovens.

Middle Eastern cooking is less precise and sophisticated than the cuisines of China and Japan and timing is less important. Some dishes such as dolmas (stuffed vine leaves) do take time to prepare but are basically very straightforward. Many dishes are ideal for entertaining as they can be prepared well in advance and in fact improve with keeping. Generally the food is spicy but not hot, with the exception of some dishes from North Africa and the Yemen. Lamb and minced meat are the most common meats but it is only in the desert that they are consumed in large quantities. Meat is expensive and so is extended with vegetables in stews and sauces. Generally the meat and vegetables are fried or sautéed before adding liquid, which gives a darker colour and richer flavour to the dish.

The cooking fat used in the past was extremely heavy with a high saturated fat content. Alya, rendered from sheep's or lamb's tail was very popular. Today, although still used in some areas, it has been generally replaced by samma (a clarified butter usually made from buffalo milk which has a strong flavour), ordinary butter, margarine and oil. Several oils are used, including olive, cotton seed, nut, corn and sesame. Olive oil is preferred for frying fish and for the many dishes eaten cold, including mezzahs, salads, fried vegetables and some meat and fish dishes. Middle

Eastern dishes can be successfully cooked with polyunsaturated oils or monounsaturated olive oil to give the authentic flavour.

Vegetables are often eaten raw and they are only rarely boiled. Nevertheless, by parboiling, you can prepare them in the Middle Eastern way using the minimum amount of oil.

In the country, wheat, usually cracked wheat or bulghur, is the staple cereal while in the urban areas rice is the basis of the meal. Bread is always served for dipping into the food. Dried beans and peas are a traditional part of the diet, as are nuts. Many Middle Eastern pulse dishes are ideal for the diabetic diet, with their high-fibre content.

Nuts are eaten whole, often with meat or vegetables, or are ground and used to thicken sauces and soups and in stuffings. The Egyptians and Syrians use ground almonds or pine nuts while Turks and Iranians use ground walnuts. In this book it has been necessary to regulate the quantities of nuts used in composite dishes because of their very high energy and fat values.

Yoghurt is another extremely popular food in the Middle East. It is eaten with a variety of dishes including stuffed vegetables, pilaus and the delicious kebabs. These are morsels of meat, chicken or fish which are cooked on skewers over charcoal. Traditionally they were cooked in charcoal-burning clay ovens called tonir or tandir which are sunk into the ground and are similar to the tandoor ovens of northern India. In Turkey, yoghurt is used as a base for meat and vegetables and as a sauce for salads, eggs and rice. It is also used as a cooking liquid, particularly in the Lebanon, Turkey and Iran. In Greece it is often eaten with honey.

In the Middle East, as in the Far East, sweet dishes are mainly reserved for visitors and for festive occasions. They are usually milk puddings or pastries, made of extremely thin filo pastry, stuffed with nuts and served with syrup. The latter are extremely rich and not to be recommended for a healthy diet. The lovely fresh fruits from the Middle East make a better and more flavoursome finish to a meal than these heavy dishes.

Latin America

The best-known cuisine of Latin America is that of Mexico, whose greatest contribution to the culinary world is the tortilla. Mexican cooking, one of the oldest cuisines in the world, developed from the Aztec and Maya civilizations when it was simple and based on beans, chillies, tropical fruit and vegetables, and wild game and turkey. Corn was sacred to the Aztecs and was the basic ingredient of the flat unleavened tortilla bread. Chocolate was and still is the popular drink. Most foods were boiled, grilled or eaten raw as the Indians did not use fats or oils in their cooking. With the Spanish influence came lard and oil for frying as well as domestic animals to provide meat and also sugar and wheat. To a lesser extent, the French, Austrians and Italians also influenced Mexican cooking. Modern Mexican cookery still strongly resembles the cooking of the Aztecs and corn, tomatoes, beans and chillies continue to be the most important foods in the Mexican diet.

The regional differences in Mexican cooking reflect differences in geography and climate. The land varies from the dry and arid north to the grassland of the coastline and the tropical rain forests of the Yucatan Peninsula. In the northern states wheat is the staple crop and so tortillas are made from wheat flour (rather than the more common corn flour). Here the Spanish influence is the strongest. Although cattle are raised in the north, beef is consumed only on special occasions and Mexican menus are designed to make meat go a long way. In the central states, pork, poultry and goat tend to be the main meats consumed but again these are eaten with plenty of vegetables. Along the coastline, fish and shellfish are abundant though generally fish is not a popular food. In the south, the most popular dishes are spicy stews.

The Mexican pattern of eating is very different from ours. They often have five meals a day, starting with an early, small breakfast, or desayuno, of coffee and tortillas. Mid-morning, a larger breakfast, or almuerzo, of eggs, beans, chilli sauce and tortillas, is served. The main meal of the day, or comida, is served in the afternoon. This includes soup, rice or a tortilla dish, a main course of meat, poultry or fish with beans, sauces, salad, vegetables and tortillas. Fruit or a crème caramel dish finishes the meal. In the early evening a light snack meal, or merienda, of chocolate or coffee with tortillas is served, followed by supper, or cena, any time after eight o'clock. No main meal is complete without beans, either cooked and served separately or mashed and fried (refritos) and used as a garnish. Beans provide the main source of protein and fibre in Mexico. Similarly, tortillas, or variations such as tacos, tamales or enchiladas, are the main source of carbohydrate.

Corn is the staple food in most of Latin America. Consumption of red meat and fish is particularly low in Ecuador where much of the protein comes from vegetable sources; the cuisine is rather bland. In contrast, the people of Brazil have a high intake of red meat. However, as in all Latin American countries, beans are eaten at nearly every meal, the most popular traditional dish being feijoada, a combination of rice, black beans, beef or bacon, herbs, spices and vegetables.

In Latin America eating is a very social occasion. The main meal of the day can last for two or three hours and unexpected visitors are always asked to join in. Entertaining is frequent and casual and whole families will get together for evenings of eating and talking.

Thus despite the many differences in geography, climate and culture, there are many similarities in the customs and the cooking methods of the countries included in this book. These cooking methods produce meals generally acknowledged to be much healthier than those commonly prepared in the West. Because of this, recipes from those countries are ideal for people wishing to improve their eating habits and are particularly suitable for people with diabetes who should in any case already be following this type of diet.

THE RECIPES

The dishes in this book have been chosen as an introduction to foods of the Far East, Middle East and Latin America. They are both healthy and delicious and are intended for the enjoyment of everyone – not just those on a special diet. When testing the recipes with my family, and eating more than the recommended portions, I found that I lost weight and we all felt fitter than on the traditional British diet.

The dishes may be enjoyed in a variety of ways. Serve them either on their own as a snack, lunch or supper dish, or with other dishes from the same country to make a traditional authentic meal. Alternatively, prepare an international menu by serving dishes from different countries. It is surprising how successful this sort of selection can be. Japanese and Chinese dishes often go well together and, as the cuisines of Malaysia and Indonesia prove, Indian and Chinese dishes complement each other perfectly. Indian and Middle Eastern dishes also have a particular affinity and I have been successful in serving meals which have combined Mexican and Middle Eastern dishes.

When choosing menus, check the food analysis at the top of each recipe to make sure that you are getting your own personal nutritional balance right. You will not, of course, have to be quite so strict with members of the family who are non-diabetic.

If you are not accustomed to hot spices, cut down on the amount of fresh or ground ginger and chilli when making a recipe for the first time. Most of the heat in fresh chillies is in the seeds, so remove these if you prefer a milder flavour. These are the spices which give the heat. You may always add a little more after tasting or on a subsequent occasion.

Alterations in seasonings will make no difference to your nutritional balance. If there is any particular herb or spice you dislike, try substituting one of your favourites. The result will not be authentic, but may well be most enjoyable and will have your own personal touch.

Equipment

Only a few pieces of equipment are essential for the preparation of the recipes in this book:

- set of standard measuring spoons
- measuring jug
- inexpensive scales with 5 g/¼ oz markings.

A few other items are certainly useful: a food processor is a boon to anyone adopting a healthy style of eating and a pestle and mortar or coffee grinder is also beneficial. For those who make a lot of fresh stock and cook beans frequently, a pressure cooker is a great time and fuel-saver.

The recipes in this book have been tested using the minimum number of pots and pans – one of each of the following:

- 2 l/3½ pint non-stick saucepan with a lid
- 22 cm/8½ in non-stick frying pan with a lid
- 26 cm/10 in non-stick frying pan with a lid
- 2 l/3½ pint ovenproof dish
- 1.5 l/2½ pint ovenproof dish
- steamer with a lid.

Later you may like to add a wok for stir-fry dishes, a *tawa* which is a convex iron griddle for cooking Indian flat breads, or a pretty Chinese bamboo steamer-set to your kitchen equipment. All are inexpensive items if bought in Asian shops.

Weights, measures and sizes

All recipes in this book have been tested and analysed using both metric and Imperial weights. The Imperial equivalents correspond as exactly as possible to the metric. It is important, however, to follow the recipes in either the metric units or the Imperial. Do not mix the two.

The tablespoon measurement used throughout this book equals 15 ml and the teaspoon 5 ml. All spoon measurements are level. Australian users should remember that as their tablespoon has been converted to 20 ml, and is therefore larger than the tablespoon measurement used in this book, they should use 3 × 5 ml/tsp where instructed to use 1 × 15 ml/tbsp.

Vegetables and fruit are described as medium. Where no size is indicated, choose medium.

Ingredients

The recipes in this book have been chosen to include as many as possible of the foods that are recommended in the Oxford Diet Plan (*The Diabetics' Diet Book*, p 19, by Dr Jim Mann and the Oxford Diatetic Group – also in this series) to be eaten regularly in a diabetic diet. Foods recommended to be taken in moderation are used occasionally and only the very minimum amounts of oil and polyunsaturated margarine, from the list of foods to be avoided, are included.

In adapting these authentic recipes to bring them into line with the new recommendations for the dietary control of diabetes, brown rice has been substituted for white, wholemeal flour for white and fats cut to a bare minimum.

Poultry has been substituted for pork and other meats and where red meat is used, it is only in small quantities to add flavour and variety to grains, vegetables and pulses.

Minimum salt is recommended in most recipes 'to taste' but it is hoped that most cooks will gradually reduce the amounts they use until their palates have adapted to the point where they may omit it altogether. There is no added sugar, no honey or syrup and no chemical substitutes.

Of course, not every traditional dish is low in fat and high in fibre. Some recipes, particularly the curries, have a high fat content. However, since most of the exotic flavours come from herbs and spices, it is easy to reduce the fat used in cooking without spoiling the flavour. Similarly, where saturated fats such as ghee or coconut oil are traditionally used, these have been substituted with a polyunsaturated oil. Although this slightly alters the flavour of the dishes it does not detract from the overall taste and many people in fact prefer the lighter corn or sunflower oils. Where olive oil is traditionally used this has not been changed. Its distinctive flavour is part of the dish and other oils would be a poor substitute especially where eaten cold. Because it has a high monounsaturated fatty acid content, it is not considered detrimental to health. The recipes are clearly marked as to whether they have a high, medium or low fat content. Usually the recipes with a high fat content have a correspondingly low level of fibre. They should not be eaten too often. The low-fat recipes can be eaten regularly if you wish. However, one word of warning. Because of the adaptations that have had to be made, particularly regarding the type and quantity of fat used, you cannot assume that the analysis of a recipe will be correct for a similar meal eaten at a restaurant.

Fat-symbols shown on the recipes indicate:
*** high fat
** medium fat
* low fat

Ethnic ingredients

Some recipes call for special ethnic ingredients. We have ensured that those used in this book are widely available in supermarkets and health food stores.

Ata flour Indian wholemeal flour used for making chapatis. Available from Indian grocers.

Bonito flakes See Katsoubushi-kezuri.

Burghul Cracked wheat with an attractive nutty flavour. Used in a similar way to rice, hot in risotto type dishes, cold as a salad in Tabbouleh. Available from large supermarkets and health food stores.

Channa dhal Very small split peas with a nutty flavour used as a spice in Indian cookery. If unavailable, substitute ordinary split peas.

Chorizo A spicy Spanish sausage. Can be found in larger supermarkets and delicatessens.

Daikon   See mooli.

Dashi   An essential stock for use in Japanese dishes. Available from Japanese grocers and health food stores.

Ful   Large brown dried beans used in Middle Eastern cookery. Available from delicatessens, or Greek or Cypriot grocers.

Katsoubushi-kezuri (bonito flakes)   Used in Japanese cookery, they have a delicate, smoky flavour. Available from Japanese grocers or health food stores.

Konbu   Dried seaweed used in Japanese cookery. Available from Japanese grocers or health food stores.

Miso   A paste made by fermenting soy beans, essential in many Japanese dishes. Available from health food stores and Japanese grocers. As it is high in salt, no further seasoning should be used.

Mooli (daikon)   A large wild white radish readily available in Indian and Japanese shops and larger supermarkets.

Nori   Seaweed paper. Available from health food stores and Japanese grocers.

Okra (ladies' fingers)   A small pointed green pod vegetable filled with seeds. Used widely in Middle Eastern and Indian cookery. Readily available in Asian and larger greengrocers and supermarkets.

Smatana   A low-fat cultured milk which contains less than half the fat of soured cream and one-fifth the fat of double cream. Available from large supermarkets or Central European delicatessens. If it is unavailable, Greek yoghurt may be substituted.

Tacos   Crisp cornmeal shells filled with savoury mixtures – a standard Mexican dish. Ready-made taco shells are widely available in large supermarkets and delicatessens. Preferably choose a brand that contains no artificial ingredients or preservatives.

Tahini   An oily paste made from sesame seeds. Widely used in Middle Eastern cookery and available from large supermarkets and health food stores.

Tamarind   A date-like but sour fruit which gives a lemony flavour to Indian dishes. Dried tamarind blocks are available from Indian grocers.

Tofu   Fermented soy bean curd with a smooth, soft consistency. It has little flavour of its own but is used as a basis for many Japanese and Chinese dishes. It is high in protein and polyunsaturated fats and low in energy. Available from health food stores.

Tostadas (tortillas)   Thin, crisp cornbreads from Mexico, served with a variety of savoury toppings. Available from large supermarkets and health food stores. Preferably choose tostadas that contain no additives.

BASICS, SOUPS, STARTERS AND SNACKS

This selection includes basic ingredients such as stock and yoghurt which provide a good foundation to the dishes. By making your own stock instead of using stock cubes, you ensure that you are using an ingredient that is free from colourings, preservatives and flavour enhancers and is low in, or free from, added salt.

Since yoghurt features in so many recipes in Eastern and Middle Eastern dishes, it is a good idea to get into the habit of making it at home. In this way you can be sure that you are getting pure, natural low-fat yoghurt which is free from all additives.

Some dishes are enriched by the addition of either smatana (see page 00) or creamy-tasting Greek yoghurt, with about the same amount of fat as smatana.

Curd cheese, low-fat Cheddar and Labna (low-fat homemade yoghurt cheese) take the place of cream cheeses and high-fat Cheddar in the recipes. Labna is popular throughout the Arab countries, where it is usually served plain for breakfast, spread on bread or shaped into small balls with olive oil and herbs. Most Western cooks prefer to serve it either as a starter or with biscuits after a meal when it is mixed with herbs. It is quick and easy to prepare, and free of additives.

Many of the starters in this section will double as a lunch or supper dish when accompanied by a grain product such as bread or rice, or simply a baked jacket potato, perhaps preceded by a soup.

In some of the recipes, more readily available ingredients have been substituted for traditional ones. In Civeche de Guiloermo (see page 50), for instance, the dish is traditionally made with shark and red snapper – but any firm white fish is suitable.

Vegetable stock
For the easiest-to-make stock: simply strain all the water from cooked vegetables into a plastic measuring jug with a lid and refrigerate for up to four days. The markings on the jug will indicate quantities as the stock is being used. Potato water should not be stored – use it straight away. Recipes for more substantial stocks follow.

***Brown vegetable stock

Makes approximately 1 l/1¾ pints

Total recipe: 135 kcal/567 kJ, negligible carbohydrate, negligible fibre, negligible protein, 15 g fat

*225 g/8 oz mixed vegetables, cut
   into large chunks
a few parsley stalks, optional
1 bay leaf
1 clove garlic (optional)*

*1 tbsp sunflower oil
salt, to taste
8 peppercorns
1 l/1¾ pints water*

Brown the vegetables, herbs and garlic very slowly in the oil, stirring occasionally to ensure they are evenly browned. Add the seasonings and water, bring to the boil, cover and simmer very gently for 2 hours. Strain, cool and refrigerate or freeze.

Variation:
White vegetable stock

Nutrient content: negligible

Use the above ingredients excluding the oil. Put all the vegetables into a saucepan. Cover with the cold water, bring to the boil, cover and continue as above.

*Chicken stock

Nutrient content: negligible

*1 chicken carcass
chicken giblets (optional)
1 carrot, chopped
1 stalk celery, chopped*

*a few herbs, to taste
1 small onion
salt and pepper*

Break up the chicken carcass and put it into a saucepan or pressure cooker with the giblets, if using. Cover with water, add the vegetables and season with salt and pepper. Bring to the boil, cover and simmer for 2-3 hours or 35-45 minutes in a pressure cooker.

Strain and refrigerate for several hours. Skim off the fat. Refrigerate for up to 4 days or freeze.

*Fish stock

Makes approximately 1 l/1¾ pints

Total recipe: 99 kcal/412 kJ, negligible carbohydrate, negligible fibre, negligible protein, negligible fat

450 g/l lb fish trimmings (heads,
   skin and bones)
1 l/1¾ pints water
a few parsley stalks
2 stalks celery

1 bay leaf
½ tsp dried thyme
pepper and salt
150 ml/¼ pint dry white wine or
   cider

Wash the fish trimmings and put them into a saucepan with the rest of the ingredients. Bring to the boil, cover and simmer very gently for 30 minutes. Strain through a fine sieve.

Note: Fishmongers will usually give you trimmings without charge.

Dashi   *Japan*
*Japanese stock
Makes approximately 1.5 l/2½ pints

Nutrient content: negligible

1.5 l/2½ pints water
15 g/½ oz konbu (see page 26)

1 × 15 g/½ oz packet katsoubushi-
   kezuri (bonito flakes, see page 26)

Put the water into the pan with the konbu and bring to the boil. When it begins to boil, remove the seaweed. Add the bonito flakes and return to the boil. Turn off the heat. Allow the bonito flakes to sink to the bottom and strain the liquid into a jug. Use as required in recipes.

Note: If bonito flakes are unavailable a mild chicken stock could be substituted, but you would miss the flavour of the real thing.

Suk mai hai yuk tong   *China*
*Crab and corn soup
Serves 4

**Each serving: 137 kcal/575 kJ, 20 g carbohydrate, 3 g fibre,
10 g protein, 1 g fat**

600 ml/1 pint dashi (see page 26),
   or fish stock (see above), or 1
   fish stock cube dissolved in
   600 ml/1 pint water
½ tsp finely grated fresh ginger
100 g/3½ oz corn

1 tbsp cornflour
1 tbsp dry sherry
170 g/6 oz fresh crab meat or canned
   crab
1 egg white
1 spring onion, finely chopped

Put the dashi or fish stock and ginger into a saucepan and bring to the boil. Add the corn and simmer for 8-10 minutes, or until the corn is tender.
   Mix the cornflour with the sherry and set aside.
   Add the fresh crab or canned crab with its liquid and the cornflour

mixture to the soup. Simmer for 2-3 minutes, stirring constantly. Turn off the heat and cover.

Beat the egg white until it becomes a light foam and stir it into the soup. Serve in individual bowls, garnished with the spring onion.

Miso shiru   *Japan*
*Miso soup with daikon and carrots

Serves 4

Each serving: 59 kcal/248 kJ, 10 g carbohydrate, 2 g fibre, 3 g protein, 1 g fat

*10 cm/4 in strip konbu (see page 26),
    or 1 l/1¾ pints vegetable stock,
    if konbu is unobtainable
1 l/1¾ pints water
4 spring onions, finely sliced*

*1 carrot cut into matchsticks
100 g/3½ oz mooli (see page 26),
    cut into matchsticks
1 tbsp miso (see page 26)
2 tbsp sake or dry sherry*

Put the konbu and water into a large saucepan and bring to the boil. Remove the konbu. Add the vegetables and boil gently for 2 minutes. Mix a little of the soup with the miso and pour it back into the pan. Add the sake or sherry and reheat. Serve immediately.

Kenchin jiru   *Japan*
*Chicken and mushroom soup

Serves 6

Each serving: 18 kcal/75 kJ, negligible carbohydrate, 1 g fibre, 3 g protein, negligible fat

*1 l/1¾ pints dashi (see page 26),
    or chicken stock (see page 29),
    or 2 chicken cubes dissolved in
    1 l/1¾ pints water
50 g/2 oz skinned chicken breast,
    cut into matchsticks*

*85 g/3 oz button mushrooms, thinly
    sliced
2 spring onions, cut into 2 cm/¾ in
    strips*

Garnish:
4-6 sprigs watercress

Put the dashi or stock into a large saucepan, bring to the boil and add the chicken. Simmer for 3-4 minutes and then add the mushrooms and spring onions. Bring to the boil. Serve in individual bowls garnished with sprigs of watercress.

Havuc çorbasi
**Carrot soup

Turkey

Serves 6

Each serving: 64 kcal/270 kJ, 10 g carbohydrate, 3 g fibre, 2 g protein, 2 g fat

1 tsp coriander seeds
15 g/½ oz polyunsaturated
margarine
450 g/1 lb carrots, finely chopped
1 l/1¾ pints chicken stock (see
page 29), or 1 stock cube dissolved
in 1 l/1¾ pints of water

2 tbsp sifted wholemeal flour
150 ml/¼ pint skimmed milk
salt and pepper

Fry the coriander seeds for a few moments in the margarine in a non-stick saucepan. Add the carrots and fry gently together for 5 minutes. Add the stock and bring to the boil. Cover and simmer for about 1 hour, or until the carrots are very soft.

Process in a food processor or blender. Alternatively, drain and mash the carrots well, then return them to the liquid.

Mix the flour with a little of the milk to make a thin paste, then add the rest of the milk. Stir into the carrot liquid, bring to the boil and simmer gently for 3-4 minutes, stirring all the time. Season with salt and pepper.

Mercimek çorbasi
*Lentil soup

Turkey

Serves 6

Each serving: 124 kcal/519 kJ, 20 g carbohydrate, 4 g fibre, 8 g protein, 2 g fat

170 g/6 oz red lentils
1 l/1¾ pints white vegetable stock
(see page 29), or 1 stock cube
dissolved in 1 l/1¾ pints water
1 small onion, coarsely chopped
1 stalk celery, coarsely chopped
1 tbsp tomato purée
1 tsp ground cumin

1 clove garlic, crushed
1 large onion, thinly sliced
15 g/½ oz polyunsaturated
margarine
salt and pepper

Garnish:
chopped fresh parsley

Put the lentils, stock, chopped onion, celery, tomato purée, cumin and garlic into a saucepan and bring to the boil. Then lower the heat, cover and simmer for about 1 hour, until the lentils are very soft (20 minutes in a pressure cooker). Process in a food processor or blender then return to the saucepan and reheat. ➡

Sopa de frijoles negro (*above*, see page 36); Sopa de cacahuate (*below*, see page 35).

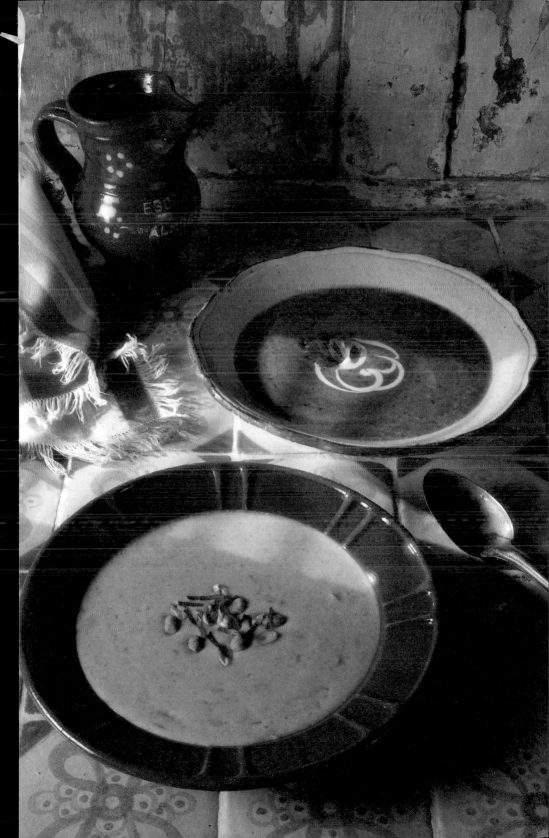

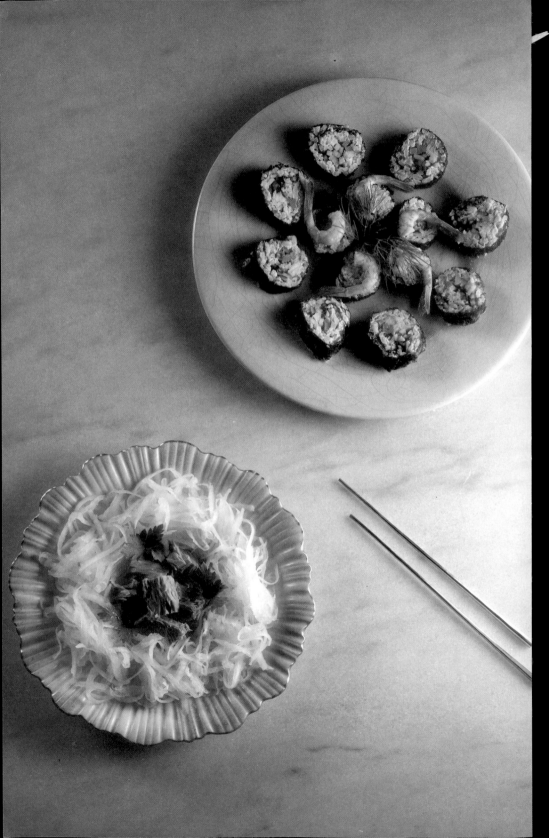

In a non-stick frying pan, gently fry the sliced onion in the margarine until just beginning to brown. Stir into the soup and season to taste. Garnish with chopped parsley.

Spanak çorbasi
*Spinach soup

Turkey

Serves 4

Each serving: 47 kcal/197 kJ, 5 g carbohydrate, 5 g fibre, 4 g protein, negligible fat

1 small carrot, chopped
1 small stalk celery, chopped
1 small onion, chopped
750 ml/1¼ pints chicken stock (see page 29), or 1 chicken or vegetable stock cube dissolved in 750 ml/1¼ pints water

225 g/8 oz fresh spinach, chopped or 115 g/4 oz chopped frozen spinach
2 tbsp fine wholemeal flour, sifted
juice of ½ lemon

In a large saucepan, boil the carrot, celery and onion in the stock until very soft. Add the spinach and simmer for 15 minutes, if fresh, 5 minutes if frozen.

Mix together the flour and lemon juice to make a thin smooth paste, adding a little cold water if necessary. Add half a cup of the soup liquid and stir well. Return the flour mixture to the soup in the pan and bring to the boil, stirring all the time. Simmer for 2 minutes and serve.

Sopa de cacahuate
***Peanut soup

Mexico

See photograph, page 33

Serves 6

Each serving: 189 kcal/794 kJ, 15 g carbohydrate, 2 g fibre, 10 g protein, 11 g fat

1 small onion, finely chopped
1 tsp sunflower oil
¾ l/1½ pints skimmed milk
20 g/¾ oz fine wholemeal flour
¼ tsp freshly grated nutmeg
grated rind of 1 lemon

100 g/3½ oz smooth peanut butter
salt and pepper

Garnish:
15 g/½ oz dry-roast peanuts
chopped fresh parsley

Maki sushi (*above*, see page 38); Tsukidash (*below*, see page 39).

Gently fry the chopped onion in the oil in a non-stick saucepan until soft. Pour in the cold milk. Sift in the flour and bring to the boil, stirring constantly. Simmer for 2-3 minutes. Stir in the nutmeg, lemon rind and peanut butter, and season with salt and pepper. Serve, garnished with the dry-roast peanuts and parsley.

Note: As it is quite high in fat, serve this soup as part of a light meal followed by a salad.

Sopa de frijoles negro   *Mexico*
*Black bean soup   **See photograph, page 33**

Serves 6

Each serving: 100 kcal/422 kJ, 15 g carbohydrate, 7 g fibre, 7 g protein, negligible fat

*150 g/5 oz dried black beans, or
   red kidney beans, soaked
   overnight*
1 small onion, chopped
1 clove garlic, finely chopped
1 tbsp tomato purée
1 bay leaf
½ tsp ground cumin
*1 l/1¾ pints chicken stock (see
   page 29), or 1 stock cube dissolved
   in 1 l/1¾ pints water*

juice of ½ a lemon

Garnish:
 2 tbsp smatana (see page 26)
 *1 tbsp finely chopped fresh coriander
   or parsley*

Drain the beans, put them into a saucepan with the onion, garlic, tomato purée, bay leaf, ground cumin and stock and bring to the boil. Boil vigorously for 10 minutes, then lower the heat, cover and simmer for 2-2½ hours (¾-1 hour in a pressure cooker) until very soft.
   Purée the mixture in a food processor or blender, or drain off the liquid and mash the beans well. Return them to the liquid and if the consistency seems too thick, add a little water. Reheat and add the lemon juice. Garnish with the smatana poured over the back of a hot teaspoon and the fresh coriander or parsley.

Sopa de verduras
*Vegetable soup

Mexico

Serves 8

Each serving: 43 kcal/179 kJ, 5 g carbohydrate, 2 g fibre, 3 g protein, negligible fat

25 g/1 oz lean back bacon, chopped
1 onion, chopped
1 clove garlic, finely chopped
1 small green chilli, finely chopped
1 red pepper, seeded and cubed
1 green pepper, seeded and cubed
1 courgette, cubed
4 tbsp tomato purée
¹/₂ tsp dried thyme

1 l/1³/₄ pints chicken stock (see page 29), or 1 chicken or vegetable stock cube dissolved in 1 l/1³/₄ pints water
200 g/7 oz sweetcorn
salt and pepper

Garnish:
1 tbsp chopped fresh parsley

Fry the chopped bacon in a large non-stick saucepan until crisp then drain on kitchen paper. Put the onion, garlic and chilli into the pan and fry until the onion is soft. Add the red and green pepper and the courgette and fry gently for 2-3 minutes. Add the rest of the ingredients except the salt, pepper and parsley and simmer for 15 minutes. Taste and season lightly. Sprinkle with parsley before serving.

Sushi
*Sushi rice

Japan

Total recipe: 403 kcal/1691 kJ, 95 g carbohydrate, 5 g fibre, 9 g protein, 2 g fat

115 g/4 oz round brown Italian rice, washed
300 ml/¹/₂ pint water
10 cm/4in piece konbu (dried seaweed, see page 26)

2 tbsp wine vinegar
large pinch of salt

Put the rice into a saucepan with the water and the konbu. Bring to the boil, cover and simmer over a very gentle heat for 40 minutes, or until all the water is absorbed and the rice is cooked. Discard the konbu. Set the pan aside, covered, for 10 minutes.

Mix together the vinegar and salt and stir into the rice. Use to make Hako sushi and Maki sushi (see page 38).

Note: Sushi is rice mixed with vinegar and shaped, either in canapé sizes with fillings or toppings, or in larger moulds. The basic rice mixture is simple and making up the shapes is creative and rewarding and an easy art to master.

Hako sushi   *Japan*
*Cup sushi
Serves 4

Each serving: 131 kcal/551 kJ, 25 g carbohydrate, 2 g fibre, 7 g protein, 1 g fat

115 g/4 oz Sushi (see page 37)
2 tbsp lemon juice
100 g/3½ oz cooked asparagus, finely chopped
50 g/2 oz smoked salmon slices

Garnish:
8 spring onions
1 lemon, cut into wedges
4 sprigs watercress

Prepare the sushi rice substituting lemon juice for the vinegar. Mix in the asparagus.
   Grease four 125 ml/4 fl oz soufflé dishes or cups lightly and line each with a piece of smoked salmon. Pack in the rice mixture, pressing it down firmly. Refrigerate.
   Just before serving, turn the mixture out on to individual plates and garnish with spring onions, lemon and watercress.

Maki sushi   *Japan*
*Rolled sushi   **See photograph, page 34**
Makes 16

Each sushi slice: 41 kcal/174 kJ, 5 g carbohydrate, 1 g fibre, 3 g protein, 1 g fat

2 sheets nori (see page 26)
1 recipe Sushi (see page 37)
85 g/3 oz smoked mackerel fillet, cut into 5 mm/¼ in thick strips
¼ cucumber, cut into 5 mm/¼ in thick strips

1 small carrot, lightly cooked and cut into 5mm/¼ in thick strips
1 tbsp creamed horseradish
1 × 50 g/2 oz can smoked oysters or a few prawns

Lay a bamboo mat or tea-towel on a work surface. Crisp the sheets of nori without scorching them by holding them briefly over a flame or hotplate. Lay one sheet on the mat, the longer edge nearest you. Spread half the rice evenly over the two-thirds of the nori closest to you, packing it firmly.

Arrange the mackerel, carrot and cucumber in a long, neat strip running horizontally across the centre of the rice. Dab on a little horseradish. Roll the mat firmly away from you, making the sushi into a very neat cylinder. Chill.

Spread the rest of the rice over the second piece of nori and roll up as before, but omitting the vegetables and fish. Chill.

Cut the chilled rolls into 2.5 cm/1 in slices and put a smoked oyster or a few prawns in the centre of the unfilled ones. Arrange attractively on a serving dish.

Tsukidash　　　　　　　　　　　　　　　　　*Japan*
***Tuna and radish salad　　See photograph, page 34

Serves 4

Each serving: 165 kcal/693 kJ, 5 g carbohydrate, 1 g fibre, 12 g protein, 11 g fat

*340 g/12 oz daikon (mooli, see
　page 26), peeled and coarsely
　grated*

*2 tsp wine or cider vinegar
1 × 200 g/7 oz can tuna, drained
　thoroughly and flaked*

Mix the daikon with the vinegar and arrange in four individual dishes. Pile the tuna in the centre.

Wafuu maa-boo dofu　　　　　　　　　　　　　*Japan*
***Mushrooms with tofu dressing

Serves 4

Each serving: 91 kcal/382 kJ, 5 g carbohydrate, 3 g fibre, 6 g protein, 6 g fat

*340 g/12 oz mushrooms
1 carrot, thinly sliced
2 tbsp sesame seeds
225 g/8 oz block tofu (see
　page 26)
1 tsp dry sherry*

*2 tsp concentrated unsweetened
　apple juice
pinch of salt*

*Garnish:
chopped fresh parsley*

Grill the mushrooms for 2-3 minutes on each side. Cut them into thin slices the same size as the carrots and put them into a bowl. Boil the carrots lightly until cooked but still crisp. Drain and add to the mushrooms.

Fry the sesame seeds in a heavy-based ungreased frying pan until they begin to pop, shaking and stirring constantly. Cool and grind to a powder in a coffee grinder or with a pestle and mortar.

Put the tofu, ground sesame seeds, sherry and apple concentrate into a food processor or liquidizer and process until smooth, adding enough water to make a thick, smooth paste. Add a little salt to taste. Pour over the mushrooms and stir together. Sprinkle over the parsley.

Imli chatney   *India*
*Tamarind chutney

Serves 8

Each serving: 61 kcal/258 kJ, 10 g carbohydrate, 1 g fibre, 2 g protein, 1 g fat

25 g/1 oz sultanas
100 g/3½ oz dried tamarind (see page 26), broken into pieces
1 small onion, grated
1 carrot, grated
1 tsp ground cumin
1 tsp grated fresh ginger

Cover the sultanas with water, bring them to the boil and set aside.

Cover the tamarind with boiling water and allow to soak until the water is cool. Knead and squeeze the pulp away from the seeds, until the fruit is dissolved in the water, then rub through a sieve. Drain the sultanas and mix with the sieved pulp, onion, carrot, cumin and grated ginger. The consistency should not be very thick. Thin with a little water if necessary.

The chutney may be kept in the refrigerator for up to a week.

RAITA   *India*
*Yoghurt sauce

Aloo raita
Potato in yoghurt sauce

Total: 526 kcal/2211 kJ, 95 g carbohydrate, 3 g fibre, 28 g protein, 6 g fat

340 g/12 oz potatoes, boiled in their skins
½ tsp cumin seeds
salt, to taste
½ tsp paprika
¼ tsp black pepper
450 ml/¾ pint low-fat yoghurt (see page 45)

Boil the potatoes in their skins until soft when pierced with a knife. Drain, peel and cool. Dice the potatoes. Put the cumin seeds into a thick ungreased frying pan and toast over a moderate heat until they begin to change colour. Beat the salt and spices into the yoghurt and mix in the cooled potatoes. Leave to stand for about 1 hour before serving.

Dhania raita
***Walnut and coriander in yoghurt sauce

Total: 520 kcal/2185 kJ, 35 g carbohydrate, 3 g fibre, 30 g protein, 31 g fat

450 ml/¾ pint low-fat yoghurt (see page 45)
1 small bunch fresh coriander
½ green chilli, seeded and minced
pinch of salt
50 g/2 oz shelled walnuts, finely chopped

Mix all the ingredients together. Leave to stand for about 1 hour before serving.

Note: Raitas are cooling side dishes eaten with hot Indian dishes. They are nutritious when eaten with pulses and grains as a protein contribution to the diet.

Betigan meshwi
***Aubergine caviar
Middle East

Serves 4

Each serving: 41 kcal/173 kJ, 5 g carbohydrate, 3 g fibre, 1 g protein, 2 g fat

450 g/1 lb aubergines
2 tsp olive oil
1 clove garlic, crushed
juice of ½ lemon
1 tbsp chopped fresh parsley
salt and pepper

Grill the aubergines, turning occasionally, until the skins are charred. Cut them open and scoop out the flesh. Put all the ingredients into a food processor and process briefly. Alternatively, mash the aubergine flesh and beat in the rest of the ingredients. Serve at room temperature with wholemeal pitta bread.

Biber salatasi
***Cold grilled peppers
Middle East

Serves 4

Each serving: 63 kcal/264 kJ, 5 g carbohydrate, 2 g fibre, 2 g protein, 4 g fat

3 green peppers
3 red peppers
black pepper
Dressing:
1 clove garlic, crushed
1 tbsp olive oil
1 tbsp lemon juice
salt (optional)
pepper

Grill the peppers until they are dark brown on all sides. Put them in a polythene bag for 10-15 minutes. Remove them one at a time and pull their skins off gently. Cut each into four, lengthways. Discard the cores and seeds. Arrange the peppers in a flat serving dish, alternating the colours.

Make the dressing: mix the garlic, oil, lemon juice and salt if using. Brush the dressing over the peppers and sprinkle generously with freshly ground black pepper. Serve cold.

Peynir salatasi   *Middle East*
***Cucumber with feta cheese dressing

Serves 4

Each serving: 103 kcal/433 kJ, 5 g carbohydrate, 1 g fibre, 5 g protein, 8 g fat

1 cucumber
1 small Spanish onion
100 g/3½ oz feta cheese, cubed
2 tsp olive oil

juice of ½ lemon
1 tsp chopped fresh oregano, or
  ½ tsp dried

Slice one quarter of the cucumber and one quarter of the onion very thinly and arrange around the edge of a flat serving dish, alternating the cucumber and the onion.

Cube the rest of the cucumber and chop the onion. Mix with the feta cheese, olive oil, lemon juice and oregano and pile into the centre of the serving dish.

Falafel   *Egypt*
**Chick pea balls

Makes 32

Each chick pea ball: 27 kcal/115 kJ, 5 g carbohydrate, 1 g fibre, 1 g protein, 1 g fat

225 g/8 oz chick peas, soaked
  overnight
1 onion
1 clove garlic
1 tbsp chopped fresh parsley
1 tsp ground coriander

1 tsp ground cumin
½ tsp turmeric
½ tsp baking powder
salt and pepper
about 200 ml/7 fl oz water
2 tsp sunflower oil, for frying

Drain the chick peas, cover with fresh water and bring to the boil. Boil vigorously for 10 minutes, then lower the heat, cover and simmer for about 1½ hours (30-40 minutes in a pressure cooker) until they are tender.

Drain, reserving the liquid, and put them into a food processor with all the other ingredients and a little of the water. Process to a very thick paste, adding a little more of the water from time to time until the desired consistency is reached. Chill.

Form into 2.5 cm/1 in balls and flatten each a little. Heat 1 tsp of the oil in a large non-stick frying pan and fry the falafel until crisp and brown.

Turn each, adding another teaspoon of oil if required and brown the other side.

Serve in wholemeal pitta bread pockets with salad and a yoghurt dressing, or omit the pitta and serve with a salad or unsweetened pickle of your choice.

Hummus bi tahini
**Chick pea purée

Middle East

Serves 6

Each serving: 78 kcal/328 kJ, 10 g carbohydrate, 3 g fibre, 4 g protein, 3 g fat

100 g/3½ oz chick peas, soaked for
  24 hours
25 g/1 oz tahini (see page 26)
1 small clove garlic, crushed
juice of 1 lemon
about 5 tbsp cold water
salt, to taste

Garnish:
paprika, a few whole chick peas and
  chopped fresh parsley

Drain the chick peas, cover with fresh water and bring to the boil. Boil vigorously for 10 minutes then lower the heat and simmer for 3-4 hours (1-1½ hours in a pressure cooker) until they are very soft. Drain and set a few aside for a garnish.

Process the rest of the chick peas with the tahini, garlic and lemon juice in a food processor or blender until quite smooth, adding enough cold water to make a thick, loose paste. Season lightly. Alternatively, crush and pound the chick peas in a pestle and mortar or strong bowl with the end of a rolling pin and beat in the rest of the ingredients a little at a time. Season to taste.

Tip into a bowl and garnish with paprika, the reserved chick peas and a little parsley. Serve as a dip with raw vegetables or with wholemeal pitta bread.

Kousa mahsi ma'ah
al-balah wa al-louz
**Courgettes stuffed with dates and nuts

Middle East

Serves 4

Each serving: 77 kcal/323 kJ, 10 g carbohydrate, 3 g fibre, 2 g protein, 4 g fat

4 medium or 2 large courgettes,
  halved lengthways
1 tsp sunflower oil
1 small onion, finely chopped
1 clove garlic, finely chopped

100 g/3½ oz mushrooms, chopped
50 g/2 oz dates, chopped
25 g/1 oz hazelnuts, coarsely
  chopped
1 tsp tomato purée

Heat the oven to 200°C/400°F/Gas 6. Steam the courgettes until they are just soft then scoop out the flesh leaving a 5 mm/¼ in 'boat'. Chop the flesh and set it aside.

Heat the oil in a non-stick pan and gently fry the onion and garlic until soft. Add the mushrooms, dates, hazelnuts, tomato purée and chopped courgettes. Mix and cook over a medium heat for 2-3 minutes.

Lay the courgette halves in a lightly greased dish and fill with the mixture. Bake for 15-20 minutes.

Dolmas
**Stuffed vine leaves

Middle East

Serves 10

Each portion: 103 kcal/435 kJ, 15 g carbohydrate, 2 g fibre, 3 g protein, 3 g fat

Filling:

1 large onion, finely chopped
1 tbsp olive oil
150 g/5 oz long-grain brown rice
225 ml/8 fl oz water
50 g/2 oz currants
2 tbsp chopped fresh parsley
2 tbsp chopped fresh mint
1 tsp allspice

25 g/1 oz pine nuts or chopped almonds
salt and pepper

1 × 225 g/8 oz package vine leaves
1 lemon
2-3 cloves garlic

Make the filling: gently fry the onion in the oil until soft. Add the rice and water and bring to the boil. Cover and simmer for 15-20 minutes until the water is absorbed. Add the currants, parsley, mint, allspice, nuts and salt and pepper. Set aside to cool.

Heat the oven to 150°C/300°F/Gas 2. Rinse the vine leaves in cold water and drain them on a wire rack. Spread them out on a work surface, shiny side down. Put 1 teaspoon of the filling on the stalk ends of the leaves. Fold over the sides and roll up to make little packets 5 × 2 cm/2 × ¾in.

Cut the zest from the lemon into fine strips, then cut the lemon into wedges.

Arrange the dolmas close together in layers in a pan, tucking in slivers of garlic and strips of lemon zest here and there. Pour over boiling water to reach the top of the dolmas. Cover closely with foil and weight down with a plate to prevent them from unrolling.

Cook in the oven for 1½-2 hours until the liquid is absorbed and the leaves and filling are tender. Cool and serve at room temperature with the lemon wedges.

Note: Any surplus can be frozen for future use.

*Low-fat yoghurt

In the three methods given here, the ingredients are identical and the results will be similar. If you use the precise method, using a thermometer or microwave probe and electric yoghurt maker, you will get a consistently high quality but, with a little practice, the simpler methods produce excellent results. Whichever method you choose, make sure that all your equipment is spotlessly clean. The longer the yoghurt ferments, the more acid the flavour.

Makes about 600 ml/1 pint yoghurt

Total: 256 kcal/1076 kJ, 40 g carbohydrate, 0 g fibre, 26 g protein, 1 g fat

568 ml/1 pint long-life (UHT) skimmed milk or fresh skimmed milk, boiled and cooled

1 tbsp dried skimmed milk powder
1 tbsp live low-fat plain yoghurt or yoghurt from your last batch

Method 1

Heat the milk to 43°C/110°F. Whisk in the dried milk and the yoghurt and pour into jars of an electric yoghurt maker or wide-mouth vacuum jug and leave undisturbed for 4-6 hours. Transfer to the refrigerator until ready to use.

Method 2

Heat the milk in a microwave oven with the probe temperature set at 41°C/106°F and proceed as in method 1.

Method 3

Heat the milk until it feels quite warm but definitely not hot to the finger. Stir the milk before testing. Pour into a warmed bowl and whisk in the dried milk and the yoghurt. Cover the bowl and wrap in a towel. Leave, undisturbed overnight, in a warm draught-free place – airing cupboard, boiler or near a cooker. Transfer to the refrigerator until ready to use.

Labna   *Middle East*
*Low-fat yoghurt cheese

Makes 325 g/11½ oz

Total: 516 kcal/2165 kJ, 60 g carbohydrate, 0 g fibre, 58 g protein, negligible fat

Make up a double quantity of the recipe for Yoghurt (see above) but stir in 2 tablespoons of dried skimmed milk powder per 568 ml/1 pint and, if liked, a little salt. When the yoghurt is set, chill for several hours in the refrigerator. Line a sieve with muslin and pour in the yoghurt. Tie the cloth in a bundle and hang over a bowl to drain overnight. Save the whey for use in wholewheat scones, sauces and soups. Use instead of curd cheese or cream cheese or make Labna balls (see below).

Labna balls   *Middle East*
*Yoghurt cheese balls   See photograph, page 51

Serves 4

Each portion: 129 kcal/541 kJ, 15 g carbohydrate, 0 g fibre, 14 g protein, negligible fat

325 g/11½ oz Labna (see above)
paprika or chopped fresh mint,
*   parsley, chives, thyme or any*
*   fresh herbs*

Make the labna into 16 balls by rolling in the palms of the hands. Leave uncovered in the refrigerator for several hours to dry out.

Roll the labna balls in paprika or serve plain, sprinkled with chopped fresh herbs of your choice.

Labna balls may be covered with olive oil after drying in the refrigerator, sealed and kept for several days in a cool place. Be sure to drain them well on kitchen paper before serving to remove excess oil.

Ensalada de mélon   *Mexico*
*Melon salad   See photograph, page 51

Serves 4

Each serving: 73 kcal/306 kJ, 10 g carbohydrate, 2 g fibre, 2 g protein, 3 g fat

Dressing:
115 ml/4 fl oz smatana (see page 26)   *1 small round lettuce*
*   or Greek yoghurt*   *1 small melon, skinned and thinly*
2 tsp olive oil   *   sliced*
2 tsp grated horseradish
pinch of chilli powder   Garnish:
1 tbsp fruit or wine vinegar   *50 g/2 oz grapes, halved and*
                                            *   seeded*

Make the dressing: beat together the smatana, oil, horseradish, chilli powder and vinegar.

Tear the lettuce and use it to line a round platter. Arrange the melon slices on top in the shape of a wheel. Pour over the dressing and garnish with the grapes.

Ensalada tropical
*Tropical salad

Serves 4

Each serving: 55 kcal/231 kJ, 15 g carbohydrate, 2 g fibre, 1 g protein, 0 g fat

*1 dessert apple, cored and finely
  sliced
juice of 1 lime
½ cucumber, finely sliced
½ small pineapple, skinned and*

*finely sliced, or 1 × 400 g/
  14 oz can of unsweetened
  pineapple in fruit juice, drained
½ tsp mild chilli powder, or to
  taste*

Toss the apple in a little of the lime juice to prevent discoloration.

Arrange the cucumber and fruit attractively on a plate. Mix the chilli powder with the remaining lime juice and pour it over the salad. Serve chilled.

Frijoles antojitos
**Bean dip

Makes 250 g/9 oz

Total: 269 kcal/1130 kJ, 30 g carbohydrate, 14 g fibre, 20 g protein, 8 g fat

*150 g/5 oz cooked red kidney beans
  (see page 36), or ½ × 400 g/14
  oz can, drained
50 g/2 oz curd cheese
2 tsp tarragon vinegar
1 clove garlic, crushed*

*½ tsp curry powder
½ tsp dried oregano
½ tsp ground coriander
½ green chilli or ¼ tsp chilli powder
1 small onion, chopped
25 g/1 oz canned red pimiento*

Put all the ingredients into a food processor or blender and process until smooth, or mash the beans, beat in the curd cheese and stir in the rest of the ingredients. Chill before serving.

Frijoles negros con chorizo
**Black beans with chorizo

Serves 4

Each serving: 201 kcal/844 kJ, 20 g carbohydrate, 11 g fibre, 14 g protein, 7 g fat

*50 g/2 oz chorizo (see page 25),
  skinned and chopped
1 small onion, chopped
1 clove garlic, finely chopped
170 g/6 oz cooked black beans or*

*red kidney beans (see page 36),
  or 2 × 400 g/14 oz cans
salt, to taste
15 g/½ oz grated Parmesan
  cheese*

▶

Fry the chorizo in a non-stick pan until the fat runs. Add the onion and garlic and fry gently with the lid on until they are soft. Drain the beans, reserving the liquid, and mash them slightly into the onion mixture. Add enough of the bean liquid to make a pleasantly thick consistency. Season, reheat and put into a serving dish.

Sprinkle with Parmesan cheese and serve with a green salad and hunks of wholemeal bread.

Tortas   *Mexico*
**Filled rolls

Serves 4

Each serving: 280 kcal/1175 kJ, 40 g carbohydrate, 12 g fibre, 15 g protein, 8 g fat

4 large wholemeal rolls
50 g/2 oz chorizo (see page 25),
*   skinned and finely chopped*
½ recipe Frijoles refritos (see
*   page 90)*

2 tomatoes, sliced
a few lettuce leaves, shredded
4 tbsp smatana (see page 26) or
*   Greek yoghurt*

Heat the rolls, cut into halves and remove part of the crumb.

Mix the chorizo with the frijoles and warm through. Divide the bean mixture between the rolls, top with the tomatoes, lettuce and smatana. Replace the lids and serve immediately.

Salsa de jitomates   *Mexico*
*Tomato sauce

Total 750 ml/1¼ pints: 209 kcal/878 kJ, 30 g carbohydrate, 9 g fibre, 13 g protein, 5 g fat

1 tsp sunflower oil
1 onion, finely chopped
1 clove garlic, crushed

2 × 400 g/14 oz cans tomatoes,
*   chopped*
2 tbsp tomato purée
1-2 green chillies, finely chopped

Heat the oil in a non-stick saucepan. Add the onion and garlic, cover and fry gently for 5-7 minutes, until the onion is soft. Add the chopped tomatoes with their juice, the tomato purée and chillies. Bring to the boil, lower the heat and simmer, uncovered, for 15-20 minutes until the sauce becomes a little thick. Alternatively, put all the ingredients, with the exception of the oil, in a food processor or blender and process briefly; the texture should not be too smooth. Heat the oil in the saucepan, add the processed ingredients, bring to the boil, lower the heat and simmer, uncovered, for 15-20 minutes.

Salsa guacamole
***Avocado sauce

Mexico

Serves 4-6

Each serving for 4: 118 kcal/495 kJ, 5 g carbohydrate, 1 g fibre, 3 g protein, 10 g fat
Each serving for 6: 79 kcal/330 kJ, 3 g carbohydrate, 1 g fibre, 2 g protein, 7 g fat

1 ripe avocado, peeled with stone removed
100 ml/3½ fl oz smatana (see page 26) or Greek yoghurt

1 green chilli
grated rind and juice of ½ orange
salt and pepper

Put all the ingredients into a food processor or blender and process until smooth. Alternatively, mash the avocado well and then beat in the rest of the ingredients.

Serve with steamed fish, chicken or as a dip with raw vegetables or taco chips.

Note: This recipe offers a way of extending avocado (with its high-fat content) so that it may be enjoyed as an occasional treat. Make the dish just before serving because an avocado, once cut, is inclined to discolour. If you must keep it, leave the stone in the sauce, cover closely with cling film and refrigerate. It will also keep quite successfully for a short time in a freezer. Defrost just before serving.

Tostadas
*Cornbread open sandwiches

Mexico

Serves 4

Each serving: 84 kcal/351 kJ, 15 g carbohydrate, 1 g fibre, 4 g protein, 2 g fat

1 tsp sunflower oil
1 small chicken breast, skinned, boned and cut into strips
2 spring onions, finely sliced
115 ml/4 fl oz Salsa de jitomates (see page 48)

4 tostadas (see page 27)
a little shredded lettuce
4 tbsp Greek yoghurt

Garnish:
1 tomato, cut into 4 slices

Heat the oven to 180°C/350°F/Gas 4. Heat the oil in a non-stick pan and fry the chicken until it is browned. Add the spring onions and the Salsa de jitomates and simmer for 2-3 minutes.

Heat the tostadas in the oven for 4-5 minutes. Spoon on the hot chicken mixture and top with the lettuce and 1 tablespoon of yoghurt on each. Garnish with a slice of tomato. Serve hot.

Tacos
**Stuffed crisp cornbreads

Mexico

Serves 6

Each serving: 139 kcal/584 kJ, 20 g carbohydrate, 5 g fibre, 7 g protein, 5 g fat

6 taco shells (see page 26)
½ recipe Frijoles refritos (see page 90)
6 tbsp Salsa de jitomates (see page 48)

a little shredded lettuce
50 g/2 oz low-fat Cheddar cheese, grated

Heat the oven to 180°C/350°F/Gas 4. Arrange the taco shells on a baking tray and heat them in the oven for 4-5 minutes. Heat the frijoles and salsa de jitomate.

Put one-sixth of the frijoles into each shell. Add a little lettuce, 1 tablespoon of the sauce and top with grated cheese. Serve immediately.

Civeche de Guiloermo
**Marinated fish

Mexico

Serves 5

Each serving: 137 kcal/577 kJ, negligible carbohydrate, 1 g fibre, 16 g protein, 7 g fat

450 g/1 lb firm white fish, skinned, boned and diced
juice of 4-5 lemons
1 small onion, finely chopped
2 tomatoes, skinned, seeded and chopped

6 green olives, stoned and chopped
1 green chilli, minced
1 tbsp chopped fresh coriander or parsley
2 tbsp olive oil
lettuce leaves for serving

Put the fish into a glass bowl and add enough lemon juice to cover it completely. Cover and leave in the refrigerator overnight.

Two or three hours before serving, drain off the lemon juice and stir in the rest of the ingredients. Refrigerate until ready to serve. Serve on a bed of lettuce leaves.

Ensalada de mélon (*above*, see page 46); Labna balls (*centre*, see page 46); Tacos (*below*).

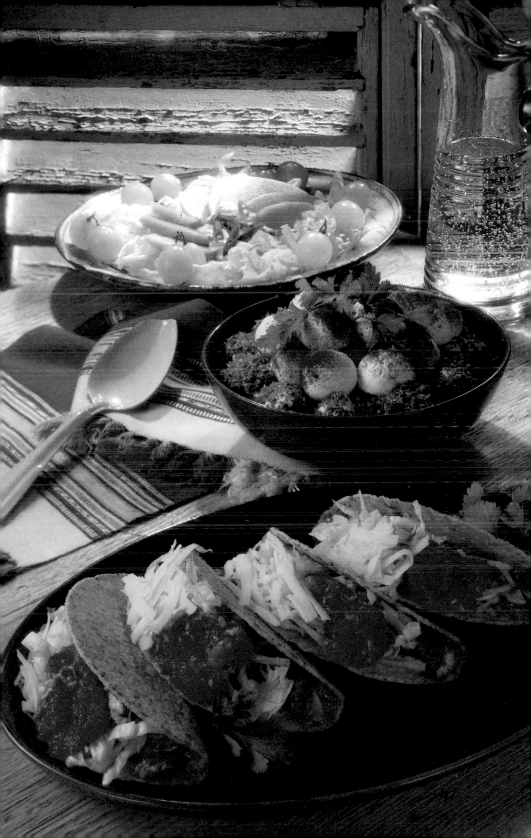

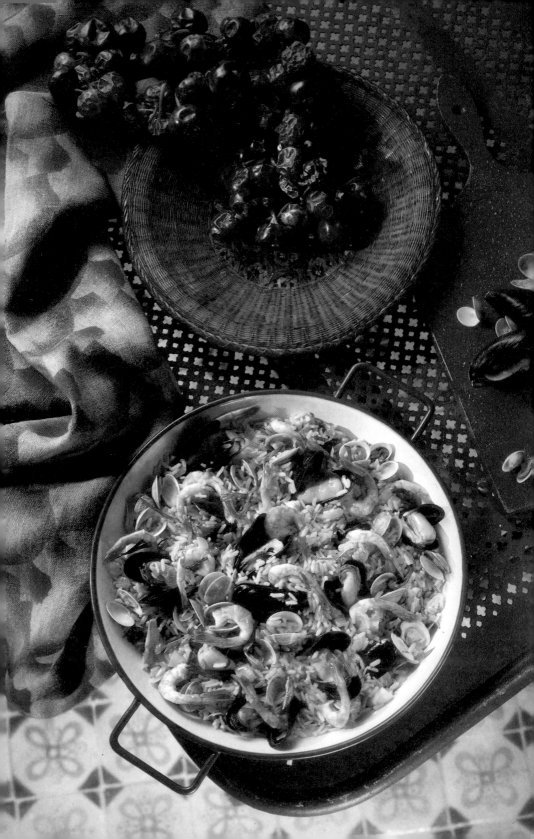

MAIN DISHES

Fish, which is low in fats, makes an excellent food for a diabetic diet. The oils found in oily fish are thought to have a positive effect on health and to contribute to the lowering of cholesterol.

Low-fat chicken and turkey are included in most of the meat dishes and, where red meat is used, it is generally in small quantities, well padded-out with other ingredients, such as burghul (cracked wheat) which is available in healthfood shops. The basis of many dishes in the Lebanon, burghul is excellent for extending meat and complementing the animal protein.

Several recipes include tofu, a fermented soybean curd which is a cholesterol-free protein food, high in polyunsaturates and low in calories and salt. Tofu can be bought in healthfood shops and has a very limited storage life. If it's not readily available, try a tofu mix which is available from Chinese grocers and some healthfood shops. This will keep indefinitely and can be made up at home in minutes, as directed on the packet.

SEA FOOD

Hai yuk sun chow fan   *China*
*Fried rice with crab and bamboo shoots

Serves 4 as part of an oriental meal

Each serving: 288 kcal/1208 kJ, 50 g carbohydrate, 3 g fibre, 14 g protein, 5 g fat

*225 g/8 oz round-grain Italian
  brown rice*
1 tbsp sunflower oil
4 spring onions, finely chopped

1 clove garlic, finely chopped
200 g/7 oz crab meat
*100 g/3½ oz canned bamboo shoots,
  cut into matchsticks*
2 tbsp light soy sauce

Boil the rice according to the packet instructions, drain and leave for several hours to dry out completely.

Heat the oil and stir-fry the onions and garlic for 1-2 minutes. Add the rice and stir-fry until heated through. Add the rest of the ingredients and stir-fry until very hot.

This will keep very well in a warm oven while you prepare vegetable dishes to accompany it.

Arros con mariscos (see page 54).

Arros con mariscos
*Rice with shellfish

See photograph, page 52   *Mexico*

Serves 4

Each serving: 325 kcal/1364 kJ, 50 g carbohydrate, 3 g fibre, 21 g protein, 6 g fat

Fish stock:
340 g/12 oz whole prawns
1 small onion, chopped
1 bay leaf
1 small carrot

450 g/1 lb mussels, cleaned and
  bearded

450 g/1 lb clams or cockles,
  cleaned
1 onion, finely chopped
1 clove garlic, finely chopped
1 green chilli, seeded and chopped
1 tbsp olive oil
225 g/8 oz long-grain brown rice,
  washed
1 tbsp fresh coriander, chopped

Make the fish stock: remove the heads and shells from the prawns. Set the prawns aside and put the heads and shells into a saucepan with the small onion, bay leaf and carrot. Cover with water and bring to the boil, then cover and simmer for 15 minutes. Strain into a large saucepan, discarding the shells.

Add the mussels and clams to the saucepan and bring to the boil. Cook, removing the shellfish with a slotted spoon as they open, and discard any which do not open. Remove one shell from each fish and discard. Set the fish aside in their half shells. Strain the liquid through a sieve lined with kitchen paper into a measuring jug. There should be 500 ml/17 fl oz. If there is too little, add water. Set aside.

Gently fry the onion, garlic and chilli in the olive oil until the onion is soft. Add the rice and prawn stock. Bring to the boil, cover and simmer for about 40 minutes, or until the rice is cooked and the liquid absorbed. Fluff rice with a fork, add the coriander, mussels in their half-shells, clams and prawns. Reheat and serve immediately.

Note: Make sure all shellfish is very fresh. The mussels and clams should be tightly closed. If they are open a little, give them a sharp tap on a firm surface. If they do not then close, discard them.

Camarones Acapulqueños
*Acapulco prawns

Mexico

Serves 4

Each serving: 74 kcal/312 kJ, 5 g carbohydrate, 2 g fibre, 11 g protein, 2 g fat

450 g/1 lb cooked prawns in their
  shells
1 small carrot

1 small stalk celery
½ bay leaf

1 clove garlic, crushed
2 tbsp chopped fresh parsley
1 tsp polyunsaturated margarine
225 g/8 oz tomatoes, skinned and

chopped or 1 × 400 g/14 oz can,
drained
2 tbsp tomato purée
pepper

Leave 4 whole prawns for garnish, peel the rest and set them aside. Put the heads and shells into a small saucepan with the carrot, celery and bay leaf and just cover with water. Bring to the boil, cover and simmer for 20 minutes. Strain into a clean saucepan, discarding the shells. Boil briskly to reduce the stock to 150 ml/¼ pint and set aside.

Gently fry the garlic and parsley in the margarine for a few moments. Add the tomatoes and simmer for about 15 minutes until almost all the liquid has evaporated. Stir in the tomato purée, the prawn stock, and a little pepper. Bring to the boil and add the prawns.

Serve in individual dishes on plain boiled brown rice or, less authentically, wholemeal pasta. Garnish with the reserved prawns.

FISH

Tsing yue I
*Steamed cod

China

Serves 4

Each serving: 96 kcal/403 kJ, negligible carbohydrate, negligible fibre, 18 g protein, 2 g fat

4 × 100 g/3½ oz cod fillets
1 clove garlic, finely chopped
1 tsp sesame oil

1 tbsp light soy sauce
1 tbsp grated fresh ginger
2 spring onions, finely chopped

Arrange the cod fillets on greaseproof paper in a steamer. Cover, place over boiling water and steam for 5-7 minutes, or until the fish is white and flakes with a fork. Remove to a heated serving dish.

Gently fry the garlic in the sesame oil, add the soy sauce and ginger and pour over the fish. Sprinkle over the chopped spring onion. Serve immediately.

Tsing yue II
***Steamed mackerel

See photograph, page 61

China

Serves 4

Each serving: 299 kcal/1256 kJ, 5 g carbohydrate, 1 g fibre, 24 g protein, 21 g fat

2 × 450 g/1 lb mackerel, scaled and
cleaned

3 tbsp light soy sauce

1 tbsp grated fresh ginger
1 tbsp wine vinegar

2 dried Chinese mushrooms, soaked
  for 30 minutes
4 spring onions, cut into shreds

Leave the heads and tails on the fish. Score the skin in diagonal cuts about 5 cm/2 in apart. Lay the fish in a dish long enough to accommodate them which will fit inside a wok or baking tin.

Mix together the soy sauce, ginger and vinegar and pour it inside and over the fish. Set aside for 30 minutes. Slice the mushrooms and put on top of the fish with the spring onions. Put the dish on a rack in the wok or baking tin. Pour sufficient water into the wok to come up to the rack. Cover, bring to the boil and cook over a moderate heat for about 10 minutes or until the fish flakes with a fork.

Serve the steamed fish with plain boiled brown rice and a Chinese stir-fried vegetable dish.

Siu sar dine yue
China
**Grilled sardines

Serves 4

Each serving: 193 kcal/811 kJ, negligible carbohydrate, negligible fibre, 22 g protein, 10 g fat

450 g/1 lb fresh sardines, cleaned
2 tbsp light soy sauce
1 tbsp dry sherry

2 spring onions, finely chopped
1 tsp grated fresh ginger
4 tbsp water

Grill the sardines for about 3 minutes on each side, until the skin is brown and crisp.

Put the rest of the ingredients into a very small saucepan and bring to the boil. Pour the sauce over the sardines and serve immediately.

Sakana no mushi yaki
Japan
*Fish baked in foil

Serves 4

Each serving: 145 kcal/608 kJ, negligible carbohydrate, 1 g fibre, 28 g protein, 3 g fat

1 tbsp sake or dry sherry
4 × 150 g/5 oz cod, haddock or hake
  fillets
4 mushrooms

12 pine kernels
¼ lemon, cut into 4 slices
½ large carrot, cut into very thin
  rings

Heat the oven to 180°C/350°F/Gas 4. Cut four × 25 cm/10 in squares of foil. Put a little sake into the centre of each to stop the fish sticking to the foil, and place the fish on the moistened foil. Arrange the rest of the ingredients attractively over the fish. Bring the sides of the foil together and fold them over twice to make a firm seal. Seal the ends. Place on a baking tray and bake for 15 minutes. Serve hot in the foil.

Machchi kebab
*Grilled fish on skewers

India

Serves 4

Each serving: 141 kcal/594 kJ, 10 g carbohydrate, 1 g fibre, 23 g protein, 2 g fat

2 tsp grated fresh ginger
2 cloves garlic, crushed
1 tbsp ground coriander
1 tsp garam masala
juice of ½ lemon

150 ml/¼ pint low-fat plain yoghurt
  (see page 45)
25 g/1 oz sifted wholemeal flour
450 g/1 lb monkfish or any thick
  white firm fish, skinned and cut
  into 4 cm/1½ in cubes

Mix the ginger, garlic, ground coriander, garam masala, lemon juice, yoghurt and flour. Add the fish, cover and marinate for 2-3 hours in the refrigerator.

Preheat the grill and thread the fish on to four skewers. Grill briskly for 4-5 minutes on each side.

Serve with a rice, a green salad and Aloo raita (see page 40).

Masala dum machchi
**Baked fish

India

Serves 4

Each serving: 155 kcal/653 kJ, 5 g carbohydrate, 0 g fibre, 21 g protein, 5 g fat

4 × 100 g/3½ oz white fish steaks
juice of ½ lemon
1 tbsp sunflower oil
2 cloves garlic, finely chopped
1 green chilli, finely chopped

1 tsp grated fresh ginger
1 tsp cumin
2 tsp garam masala
225 ml/8 fl oz low-fat plain yoghurt
  (see page 45)

Heat the oven to 200°C/400°F/Gas 6. Arrange the fish steaks in an oven-to-table dish just large enough to take them in one layer. Rub each steak with a little lemon juice.

Heat the oil in a small saucepan and fry the garlic, chilli and ginger for 2-3 minutes. Add the cumin and the garam masala and fry for 2-3 more minutes. Add the yoghurt one spoon at a time, making sure that each spoonful is thoroughly amalgamated before adding the rest. Pour over the fish and bake in the oven for 15-20 minutes, or until the fish is opaque and flakes with a fork.

Samak masloak
Middle East
*Fish stew

Serves 4

Each serving: 201 kcal/845 kJ, 15 g carbohydrate, 10 g fibre, 28 g protein, 4 g fat

50 g/2 oz haricot beans, soaked overnight
450 g/1 lb thick coley or cod, skinned and cut into large chunks
juice of 1 lemon
15 g/½ oz polyunsaturated margarine
450 g/1 lb fresh spinach, chopped or 225 g/8 oz frozen chopped spinach

225 g/8 oz leeks, thinly sliced
1 small stalk celery, finely chopped
300 ml/½ pint fish stock (see page 29), or ½ fish stock cube dissolved in 300 ml/½ pint water
1 tsp turmeric
pepper, to taste

Garnish:
2 tbsp chopped fresh parsley

Drain the beans, cover with fresh water and bring to the boil. Boil vigorously for 10 minutes, then lower the heat, cover and simmer for 1½-2 hours. Alternatively, omit the soaking and cook the beans for 25-35 minutes in a pressure cooker. Drain.

Marinate the fish in the lemon juice for 1-2 hours.

Melt the margarine in a non-stick saucepan and gently fry the spinach, leeks and celery for 2-3 minutes. Add the stock, cooked drained beans and turmeric. Bring to the boil, cover and simmer for 15 minutes. Add the fish with the lemon juice and simmer for 7-10 minutes, or until the fish looks white and it flakes with a fork. Season with pepper to taste and garnish with parsley.

Serve with Burghul pilav (see page 114) or boiled brown rice.

Ribi
Middle East
*Fish steaks

Serves 4

Each serving: 242 kcal/1018 kJ, 10 g carbohydrate, 6 g fibre, 28 g protein, 7 g fat

4 × 115 g/4 oz white fish steaks
1 tbsp fine wholemeal flour
1 tbsp sunflower oil
2 leeks, cut into 1 cm/½ in slices
400 g/14 oz can tomatoes, drained and chopped

4 canned pimientos, sliced
150 ml/¼ pint dry white wine
pepper, to taste
2 tbsp chopped fresh parsley

2 tbsp low-fat yoghurt (see page 45)
50 g/2 oz low-fat Cheddar cheese,
  grated

Garnish:
1 lemon, cut into wedges

Heat the oven to 180°C/350°F/Gas 4. Dip the fish cutlets into the flour and fry them in the oil in a non-stick frying pan until they start to brown on each side. Put them into an oven-to-table dish large enough to accommodate them in one layer or into individual dishes.

In the same pan, fry the leeks, then add the tomatoes, pimientos and wine and simmer until the sauce is thick. Add the pepper and parsley and pour the sauce over the cutlets. Spoon over the yoghurt and sprinkle with grated cheese. Bake for 15 minutes.

Serve garnished with lemon wedges and hunks of wholemeal bread or with brown rice or vegetables of your choice.

Samak mahshi bil-firin
***Stuffed baked trout

Middle East

Serves 4

Each serving: 249 kcal/1045 kJ, negligible carbohydrate, 1 g fibre, 32 g protein, 13 g fat

15 g/½ oz polyunsaturated
  margarine
2 tbsp finely chopped fresh
  tarragon
3 spring onions, finely chopped, or
  a small handful of chives
2 tsp finely chopped fresh
  coriander
2 tbsp finely chopped fresh mint

2 tbsp finely chopped fresh parsley
juice of 1 lemon
1 tbsp oil
4 small trout

Garnish:
lemon wedges
fresh herbs

Heat the oven to 200°C/400°F/Gas 6. Melt the margarine in a small non-stick saucepan. Add all the herbs (use those which are available and substitute if necessary) and fry for 2 minutes. Add the lemon juice and set aside to cool.

Grease an ovenproof dish very lightly. Stuff the trout with the herb mixture and lay them in the dish. Brush with very little oil and bake in the oven for 15-20 minutes. Serve garnished with lemon wedges and herbs.

Pescado a la Veracruzana
**Fish in the Veracruz style

Mexico

Serves 4

Each serving: 180 kcal/755 kJ, 15 g carbohydrate, 2 g fibre, 19 g protein, 5 g fat

225 g/8 oz potatoes
1 onion, chopped
2 cloves garlic, finely chopped

1 tbsp olive oil
225 g/8 oz tomatoes, skinned and
  chopped or 1 × 400 g/14 oz can,
  drained and chopped

2 tbsp capers	pepper, to taste
10 green olives, stoned and chopped	4 × 100 g/3½ oz fillets firm white fish
1 bay leaf	

Cook the potatoes, cut into large chunks and set aside. Gently fry the onion and garlic in the oil until soft. Add the tomatoes, capers, olives, bay leaf and pepper. Bring to the boil and simmer, uncovered, for 10 minutes.

Arrange the fish in one layer in a flameproof dish, add the potatoes and pour over the sauce. Bring to the boil, cover and simmer for 10 minutes, or until the fish is tender and opaque. Alternatively, heat the oven to 200°C/400°F/Gas 6. Lay the fish in a lightly greased shallow ovenproof dish or individual gratin dishes, arrange the potatoes around the fish and cover with the sauce. Bake in the oven for 15 minutes.

Serve with plain boiled brown rice or chunks of wholemeal bread.

Pescado en jugo de naranja
**Fish in orange juice

Mexico

Serves 4

Each serving: 170 kcal/716 kJ, 5 g carbohydrate, 1 g fibre, 24 g protein, 6 g fat

1 tbsp plus 1 tsp sunflower oil	4 × 150 g/5 oz cod steaks, or other white fish
2 cloves garlic, crushed	1 onion, thinly sliced
½ tsp ground cumin	1 canned pimiento, drained and thinly sliced
½ tsp dried oregano	
juice of 2 Seville oranges, or 2 small sweet oranges plus juice of ½ lemon	Garnish:
	1 tbsp chopped fresh parsley

Mix together the tablespoon of oil, garlic, cumin, oregano and orange juice. Arrange the fish in a lightly greased ovenproof dish large enough to accommodate it in one layer and pour over the orange juice mixture. Leave to stand in a cool place for 1-3 hours.

Heat the oven to 200°C/400°F/Gas 6. Gently fry the onion in the teaspoon of oil in a non-stick pan until soft. Arrange over the fish with the pimiento. Bake in the oven for 15-20 minutes, until the fish is opaque and flakes with a fork. Sprinkle over the parsley. Serve with plain boiled brown rice or jacket potatoes.

Pescado en jugo de naranja (*above*); Tsing yue II (*below*, see page 55).
OVERLEAF: Nasi goreng (*top left*, see page 69); Yakitori (*below left*, see page 68); Shabu-shabu (*right*, see page 66).

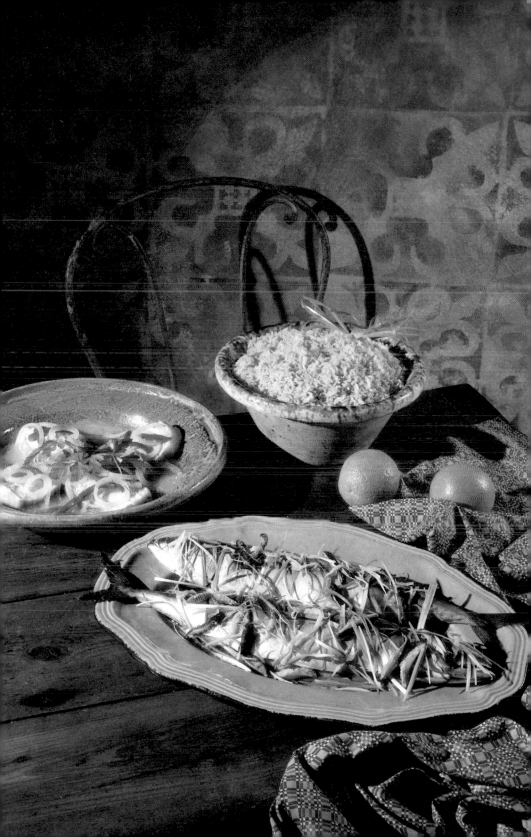

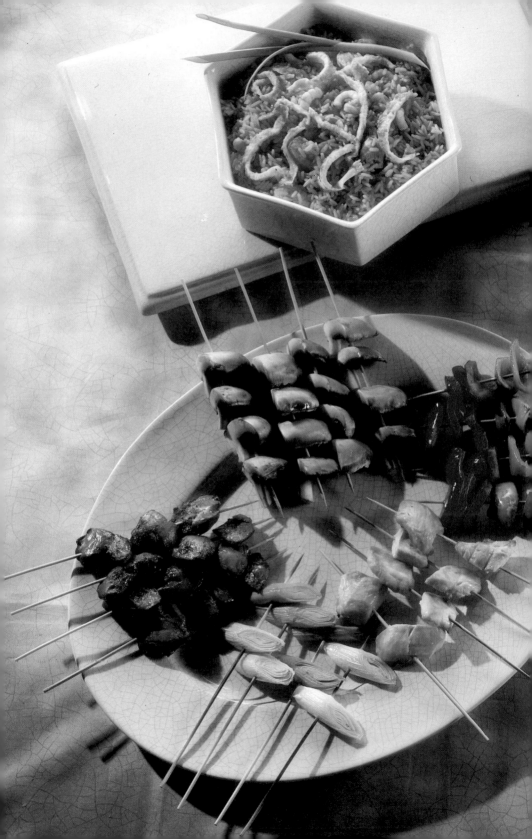

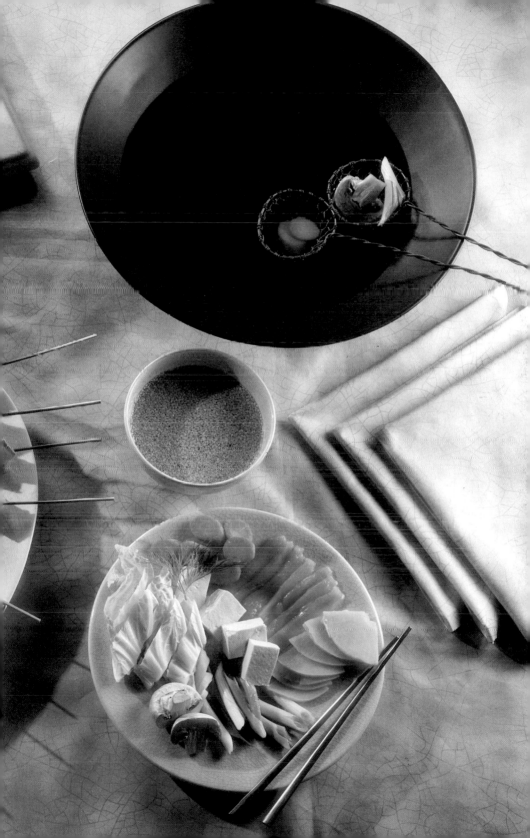

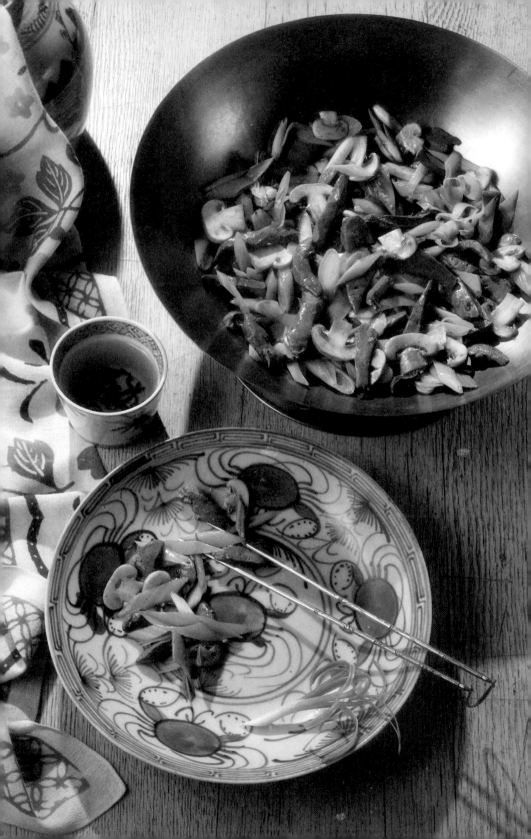

Pescado con salsa guacamole   *Mexico*
***Steamed fish with avocado sauce

Serves 4

Each serving: 204 kcal/856 kJ, 5 g carbohydrate, 1 g fibre, 23 g protein, 11 g fat

450 g/1 lb white fish fillets, skinned or steaks, unskinned

juice of ½ lemon
1 recipe Salsa guacamole (see page 49)

Sprinkle the fish with lemon juice. Line a steamer with greaseproof paper and lay the fish on the paper. Steam for about 10 minutes, or until the fish flakes with a fork. Serve hot or cold with Salsa guacamole.

POULTRY

Pan say saw   *Taiwan*
**Lee's Taiwanese shredded turkey and vegetable

Serves 4

Each serving: 244 kcal/1023 kJ, 25 g carbohydrate, 4 g fibre, 16 g protein, 9 g fat

4½ tbsp light soy sauce
1 tsp dry sherry
2 tbsp water
3 tbsp cornflour
225 g/8 oz turkey breast, cut into 4 cm × 5mm/1½ × ¼ in strips
1 carrot, cut into strips 6 cm × 5 mm/2½ × ¼ in wide
pepper, to taste
4 tsp white wine vinegar

2 tbsp sunflower oil
1 onion, chopped
200 g/7 oz mushrooms, sliced
1 × 200 g/7 oz can bamboo shoots, drained, cut into strips, 6 cm × 5 mm/2½ × ¼ in wide
450 ml/¾ pint water
50 g/2 oz shelled peas, fresh or frozen
a few drops of sesame oil

Dai suen chow yeung gone (see page 76).

Mix 2 teaspoons of the soy sauce with the sherry, water and 1 tablespoon cornflour. Add the meat and leave to soak.

Mix together 2 tablespoons cornflour, the remaining soy sauce, pepper and the vinegar. Set aside.

Heat the sunflower oil in a wok or non-stick frying pan, add the turkey and fry for 3 minutes, stirring all the time. Remove on to a plate with a slotted spoon, shaking off the excess oil.

Put the onion into the wok and fry until golden, then add the mushrooms, bamboo shoots, carrot and water. Bring to the boil, add the peas and cook for another 2 minutes. Add the meat and soy sauce mixture. Cook for 1-2 minutes stirring all the time. Sprinkle with a little sesame oil.

Serve with plain boiled brown rice.

Shabu-shabu   *Japan*
*Simmered chicken and vegetables   See photograph,
Serves 4   page 63

Each serving: 486 kcal/2042 kJ, 60 g carbohydrate, 8 g fibre, 37 g protein, 13 g fat

450 g/1 lb skinned and boned
  chicken breasts
2 large carrots, cut into rounds
4-6 Chinese leaves, cut into 6 cm/
  2½ in lengths
1 bunch spring onions, cut into
  6 cm/2½ in lengths
225 g/8 oz small button
  mushrooms
1 × 200 g/7 oz can bamboo shoots,
  drained and thinly sliced
450 g/1 lb block tofu (see page 26),
  cut into 2.5 cm/1 in squares

1 l/1¾ pints boiling chicken stock
  (see page 29), or 1 stock cube
  dissolved in 1 l/1¾ pints water

Sauce:
50 g/2 oz sesame seeds
2 tbsp lemon juice
8 tbsp light soy sauce
2 tsp finely grated fresh ginger
4 tbsp water

225 g/8 oz long-grain brown rice

Freeze the chicken lightly and, using a very sharp knife, cut it into paper thin slices. As cooking time is short it must be very thin. Arrange it attractively on a plate, cover and thaw in the refrigerator.

Boil the carrots for 3-4 minutes, then drain and cool. Arrange all the vegetables and the tofu on separate plates.

Make the sauce: put the sesame seeds in a heavy-based ungreased frying pan and cook over a medium heat until they begin to pop. Grind them in a coffee grinder or pestle and mortar. Mix with the rest of the sauce ingredients.

Boil the rice.

Set the table with the pan of boiling stock in the centre and arrange the plates of meat and vegetables around it. Give each guest a bowl of the sauce and a bowl of rice.

When all the chicken and vegetables are eaten, serve the stock as a soup.

Note: This is an Eastern version of the fondue. You will need a fondue dish, or electric frying pan, or any heatproof dish over a fairly brisk burner and fondue forks. Guests pierce pieces of chicken or vegetable and cook them in the simmering stock. The cooked food is then dipped in the sauce and eaten with the rice. All the food may be prepared 2-3 hours ahead of time, covered with cling film and refrigerated.

Domburi
Japan

**Tofu and chicken savoury mince

Serves 4

Each serving: 185 kcal/777 kJ, 10 g carbohydrate, 3 g fibre,
17 g protein, 8 g fat

450g/1 lb block tofu (see page 26)
6 Chinese dried mushrooms or fresh mushrooms, thinly sliced
1 tsp sunflower oil
1½ tsp grated fresh ginger
150 g/5 oz skinned and boned dark chicken meat, minced
115 g/4 oz carrots, cut into matchstick strips
100 g/3½ oz shelled peas, fresh or frozen
4 spring onions, finely sliced
3 tbsp light soy sauce
2 tbsp sake or dry sherry
1 egg, lightly beaten

Break up the tofu with a fork and leave to drain in a sieve. Soak the dried mushrooms, if using, in hot water for 15-20 minutes. Drain, discard the stems and slice the caps thinly.

Heat the oil in a non-stick saucepan. Add the ginger and minced chicken and fry gently until the chicken changes colour, breaking up the mince with chopsticks or a wooden fork. Add the carrots, peas and mushrooms and fry gently with the lid on for about 4-5 minutes, tossing occasionally, until the carrots are tender but still crisp. Add the tofu and the spring onions and mix gently until the tofu is heated through. Sprinkle over the soy sauce and sake. Remove from the heat and stir in the egg.

Serve with plain boiled brown rice.

Toriniku no oven yaki
Japan

*Oven baked chicken

Serves 4

Each serving: 154 kcal/646 kJ, 5 g carbohydrate, 1 g fibre, 20 g protein,
4 g fat

4 small chicken portions, skinned
2 tsp cornflour
4 tbsp shoyu or light soy sauce
4 tbsp dry sherry
1 tbsp concentrated unsweetened apple juice
2 slices unpeeled lemon, finely chopped
1 clove garlic, crushed
2 tsp grated fresh ginger

▶

Arrange the chicken, fleshy side down, in a baking dish just large enough to take the pieces in one layer. Mix together the rest of the ingredients and pour over the chicken. Leave for several hours for the chicken to absorb the flavour of the marinade.

Heat the oven to 200°C/400°F/Gas 6. Put the dish into the oven and cook for 30-40 minutes, turning the chicken pieces halfway through and basting frequently, until the juices run clear when the chicken is pierced with the point of a knife.

Serve Japanese-style with rice, or Western-style with vegetables of your choice.

Yakitori
*Chicken on skewers

Japan

See photograph, page 62

Serves 4

Each serving: 178 kcal/750 kJ, 10 g carbohydrate, 3 g fibre, 22 g protein, 5 g fat

Sauce:

2 tbsp concentrated unsweetened apple juice
115 ml/4 fl oz dry white wine
115 ml/4 fl oz shoyu or light soy sauce

a little oil, for brushing
200 g/7 oz boned and skinned chicken breasts, cut into 2.5 cm/ 1 in squares

150 g/5 oz chicken livers, cut into 2.5 cm/1 in squares
4 large mushrooms, cut into eighths
1 green pepper, seeded and cut into 2.5 cm/1 in squares
1 red pepper, seeded and cut into 2.5 cm/1 in squares
2 thin leeks, cut into short lengths

Make the sauce by mixing together the apple juice, wine and soy sauce. Pour into a tall glass. Lightly brush metal skewers with a little oil – you will need 24.

Thread the chicken on to four skewers, leaving spaces between each piece; similarly thread the liver and the different vegetables each on separate skewers.

Heat the grill, dip the skewers in the sauce and start by grilling the leeks, which will take a little longer than the rest of the skewers. Add the remaining skewers and turn, brushing with sauce as they brown.

If preferred, vegetables, chicken and liver may be mixed on the skewers, but in this case make different combinations of ingredients, for example, chicken and leek, or mushroom and peppers, so that they look interesting and attractive.

Serve with boiled brown rice.

Note: Traditionally bamboo skewers are used. They are well soaked in water to prevent them from burning.

Pad thua ngork
**Fried beansprouts

Serves 4 as part of an oriental meal

Each serving: 111 kcal/467 kJ, negligible carbohydrate, 2 g fibre, 14 g protein, 5 g fat

1 tbsp sunflower oil
3 cloves garlic, finely chopped
100 g/3½ oz turkey, cut into very
 tiny cubes
100 g/3½ oz prawns

300 g/10½ oz beansprouts
pepper, to taste
1 tbsp anchovy essence
1 tbsp light soy sauce

Heat the oil in a wok or a non-stick frying pan and fry the garlic until it is golden. Add the turkey and stir-fry for 2 minutes. Add the prawns and beansprouts and stir-fry for 1-2 minutes, until cooked but still crisp. Add the flavourings.

Nasi goreng
*Fried rice

See photograph, page 62

Serves 4

Each serving: 332 kcal/1394 kJ, 50 g carbohydrate, 3 g fibre, 18 g protein, 8 g fat

Omelette:
1 tsp sunflower oil
1 egg, beaten

Rice:
1 tbsp sunflower oil
100 g/3½ oz onion, finely chopped
2 cloves garlic, finely chopped

¼ tsp chilli powder
½ tsp Chinese shrimp sauce
100 g/3½ oz turkey, diced
2 tbsp light soy sauce
225 g/8 oz brown rice, cooked and
 drained well ahead of time
100 g/3½ oz cooked peeled
 prawns

Make the omelette: heat the teaspoon of oil in a large non-stick frying pan. Pour in the egg and cook until it is set. Set aside to cool, then cut it into thin strips.

Heat the tablespoon of oil and fry the onion and garlic with the chilli and shrimp sauce until light brown. Add the turkey and continue frying until the meat is cooked. Add the soy sauce and stir in the rice, coating each grain with the mixture. Add the prawns and stir-fry until the rice is heated through.

Serve decorated with the omelette slices with chutney, pickles, tomatoes and cucumber.

Murgh pulao
*Chicken pilau

India

Serves 4

Each serving: 401 kcal/1686 kJ, 55 g carbohydrate, 5 g fibre, 25 g protein, 10 g fat

½ × 1.8 kg/4 lb chicken, or 4 small
chicken portions, skinned and cut
into 8 pieces
3 whole green cardamom pods,
crushed
5 cm/2 in cinnamon stick
½ tsp mustard seeds
4 peppercorns
5 whole cloves
½ tsp cumin seeds

salt, to taste
15 g/½ oz polyunsaturated
margarine
225 g/8 oz onions, chopped
225 g/8 oz basmati rice, well washed
and drained
100 g/3½ oz shelled peas, fresh or
frozen
15 g/½ oz blanched sliced
almonds

Put the chicken pieces into a saucepan with the spices and salt to taste and just cover with water. Bring to the boil, cover and simmer for 10 minutes.

Melt the margarine in a large non-stick pan and fry the onions gently until golden. Lift the chicken out of the liquid with a slotted spoon and fry with the onions until it is golden. Measure the liquid from the chicken and make it up to 450 ml/¾ pint with water. Add this to the chicken with the rice, peas and almonds. Bring to the boil, cover and simmer for about 12-15 minutes until it has almost boiled dry. Remove from the heat and set aside in a warm place for 10 minutes.

Serve with a vegetable curry, and Imli chatney (see page 40) or Dhania raita (see page 41).

Murgh tandoori
**Tandoori chicken

India

Serves 4

Each serving: 215 kcal/903 kJ, 5 g carbohydrate, 0 g fibre, 33 g protein, 8 g fat

4 chicken quarters, skinned
2 tbsp lemon juice
2 tbsp tandoori mixed spice

4 tbsp low-fat plain yoghurt (see
page 45)
2 tbsp wine vinegar

The day before serving, make four parallel cuts in the flesh of each chicken quarter, almost to the bone. Pour the lemon juice over the chicken and rub well into the slits. Mix together all the other ingredients and pour over the chicken. Cover and leave overnight in a cool place, turning occasionally.

The next day, shake off the excess marinade from the chicken and grill over charcoal or under a very hot grill for 10-15 minutes on each side.

Serve sizzling hot with a vegetable curry and Pyaaz sambal (see page 107) and an Indian bread such as naan (see page 116) or chapatis (see page 115).

Auff sum sum
Israel
***Oven-fried sesame drumsticks

Serves 6

**Each serving: 222 kcal/931 kJ, 10 g carbohydrate, 2 g fibre,
17 g protein, 13 g fat**

1 egg	*70 g/2½ oz wholemeal flour*
1 tbsp sunflower oil	*pinch of salt*
4 tbsp water	*1 tsp paprika*
70 g/2½ oz sesame seeds	*6 chicken drumsticks, skinned*

Heat the oven to 200°C/400°F/Gas 6. Beat together the egg, oil and water.
In another dish mix together the sesame seeds, flour, salt and paprika.

Dip the chicken legs into the egg mixture and then into the dry mixture
and lay them on a lightly greased baking tray. Bake in the oven for 25-30
minutes.

Serve hot or cold.

Morgh sofrito
Middle East
**Cold jellied chicken

Serves 6

**Each serving: 143 kcal/602 kJ, negligible carbohydrate, negligible fibre,
23 g protein, 5 g fat**

1.5 kg/3 lb chicken	*Garnish:*
juice of 1 lemon	*chopped fresh parsley*
1 tsp turmeric	*slices of lemon*
2 green cardamom seeds, crushed	*slices of cucumber*
300 ml/½ pint water	
salt and pepper	

Put all the ingredients into a saucepan just large enough to hold the
chicken. Bring to the boil, cover and simmer for about 1 hour until the
chicken is very tender. Check from time to time adding more water if
necessary. Allow the chicken to cool in the liquid.

Strain the stock and chill. Lift off all the fat and reheat the stock. Joint
and skin the chicken and arrange on a serving dish. Pour the liquid over
the chicken and refrigerate. As it begins to set, spoon the liquid over the
top of the chicken to glaze it.

Serve at room temperature garnished with parsley, lemon and
cucumber. Although it is not traditional, this dish would make an
attractive party dish with the boned chicken set with the jelly in a ring
mould, the centre filled with Laban salateen (see page 107).

Hav ganachov
**Chicken with vegetables

Serves 4

Each serving: 233 kcal/978 kJ, 20 g carbohydrate, 9 g fibre, 24 g protein, 7 g fat

1 large aubergine, sliced into 1 cm/ *½ in rings* *salt* *½ × 1.8 kg/4 lb chicken, jointed* *into 4, or 4 small chicken* *portions* *2 tsp sunflower oil* *1 Spanish onion, peeled and sliced* *2 courgettes, sliced* *1 green pepper, seeded and sliced* *225 g/8 oz French beans, or runner* *beans, sliced*	*2 tbsp fine wholemeal flour* *1 tsp ground cumin* *¼ tsp chilli powder* *1 bay leaf* *pepper, to taste* *2 tomatoes, skinned and sliced* Garnish: *2 tbsp chopped fresh parsley*

Put the aubergine slices into a colander and sprinkle with a little salt. Set aside for 30 minutes then rinse off the salt and drain.

Heat the oven to 180°C/350°F/Gas 4. Grill the chicken on all sides under a hot grill until golden. Set aside.

Heat the oil in a large non-stick frying pan with a lid. Fry the onion for 5 minutes and add the courgettes, peppers, aubergine and beans. Fry gently for 5-10 minutes with the lid on then stir in the flour, cumin, chilli, bay leaf, and salt and pepper to taste.

Put the vegetables into a lightly greased 2 l/3½ pint, shallow ovenproof dish. Arrange the chicken portions on top and tuck slices of tomato in between the chicken pieces. Cover the dish with a lid or foil and bake for 1 hour. Sprinkle with the parsley and serve with plain boiled brown rice.

Kabsa dighagh
*Chicken liver pilav

Serves 5

Each serving: 348 kcal/1460 kJ, 55 g carbohydrate, 4 g fibre, 14 g protein, 10 g fat

1 tbsp sunflower oil *1 onion, finely chopped* *225 g/8 oz chicken livers, diced* *25 g/1 oz almonds, chopped* *50 g/2 oz raisins*	*6 green cardamoms* *2.5 cm/2 in stick cinnamon* *285 g/10 oz Italian brown rice* *600 ml/1 pint water* *salt, to taste*

Heat the oil in a large non-stick frying pan and fry the onion until brown. Add the chicken livers and fry until they stiffen and colour. Add the rest of the ingredients, stir and bring to the boil. Cover, lower the heat and simmer for 30-40 minutes, or until the rice is cooked. Check after 20 minutes to make sure the rice is not drying out too much. Add more boiling water if necessary. Serve with a salad.

Koftit ferakh
**Chicken balls

Egypt

Serves 4

Each serving: 197 kcal/827 kJ, 15 g carbohydrate, 4 g fibre, 22 g protein, 7 g fat

115 g/4 oz wholemeal bread
225 g/8 oz cooked chicken
25 g/1 oz sunflower seeds

3 tbsp chopped fresh parsley
juice of ½ lemon
salt and pepper

Soak the bread in a little water for a few minutes. Mince the chicken. Squeeze out the bread and mix all the ingredients together. Alternatively, put all the ingredients in a food processor and process until the mixture is firm.

Take 1 teaspoon of the mixture at a time and roll into balls with wet hands. Chill.

Serve with salad and pitta bread.

Kebab
**Turkey kebabs

Israel

Serves 4

Each serving: 198 kcal/830 kJ, 5 g carbohydrate, 1 g fibre, 27 g protein, 9 g fat

2 tbsp olive oil
juice of 1 lemon
1 tsp dried oregano
1 clove garlic
pepper, to taste

450 g/1 lb thick turkey breast, cut
into 3 cm/1¼ in chunks
12 pickling onions, peeled
1 red pepper, seeded and cut into
3 cm/1¼ in chunks
1 green pepper, seeded and cut into
3 cm/1¼ in chunks

Mix together the oil, lemon juice, oregano, garlic and black pepper. Stir in the turkey and marinate 1-2 days in the refrigerator, stirring occasionally.

Blanch the onions in boiling water for 2-3 minutes. Strain and cool. Thread the peppers on to four skewers, alternating with the turkey and onions. Grill under a moderate grill or on a barbecue turning occasionally and basting with the marinade, until the turkey is thoroughly cooked, about 15 minutes in all.

Serve with brown rice pilav, wholemeal pitta bread or chunks of wholemeal bread and a green salad or vegetables.

Arroz con pollo
Latin America
*Rice with chicken

Serves 4

Each serving: 279 kcal/1171 kJ, 40 g carbohydrate, 8 g fibre, 18 g protein, 7 g fat

2 large chicken breasts, skinned and boned
1 small carrot
1 stalk celery
salt and pepper
500 ml/17 fl oz water
1 tbsp sunflower oil
1 onion
1 clove garlic
150 g/5 oz long-grain brown rice, washed and drained

225 g/8 oz shelled peas, fresh or frozen
6 olives, stoned and quartered
1 tsp dried oregano
½ tsp cumin
1 × 400 g/14 oz can tomatoes, chopped

Garnish:
1 canned pimiento, thinly sliced

Put the chicken breasts into a saucepan with the carrot, celery, salt, pepper and water and bring to the boil. Cover and simmer for 30 minutes. Drain, reserving the stock. Cool the chicken and tear it into large pieces with your hands. Set aside.

Heat the oven to 180°C/350°F/Gas 4. Heat the oil in a non-stick pan and gently fry the onion and garlic until soft. Add the rice and fry gently for 2-3 minutes, coating the grains with the oil. Add the peas, olives, oregano, cumin and tomatoes with their juice and bring to the boil.

Arrange the chicken pieces in a greased 2 l/3½ pint shallow ovenproof dish and add the rice mixture. Pour in enough of the reserved chicken stock to come up to the top of the rice. Cover with a lid or foil and bake for 1-1¼ hours or until the rice is cooked and most of the liquid is absorbed – the finished dish should be very moist. Remove the lid and garnish with the pimiento. Return to the oven for 5 minutes before serving.

Guajolote en salsa chile rojo
Mexico
**Turkey in red chilli sauce

Serves 4

Each serving: 186 kcal/780 kJ, 5 g carbohydrate, 1 g fibre, 28 g protein, 5 g fat

1 tbsp sunflower oil
1 onion, chopped
450 g/1 lb boned and skinned turkey, cut into large chunks
2 tsp mild chilli powder
2 cloves garlic, crushed

1 × 400 g/14 oz can tomatoes, chopped
2 tbsp tomato purée
½ tsp dried basil
½ tsp cumin
1 small stick cinnamon

Heat the oil in a large non-stick saucepan, add the onion and fry gently for 5-7 minutes, until soft. Add the turkey and fry until it begins to brown. Stir in the chilli and the garlic and fry for 1 minute. Add the tomatoes, tomato purée, basil, cumin and cinnamon and bring to the boil. Cover the pan and simmer gently for 30-40 minutes, until the meat is cooked and tender.

Serve with brown rice and Ejotes con jugo de lima (see page 103) or another green vegetable or salad.

Pollo con elote   *Mexico*
**Chicken with corn

Serves 4

Each serving: 250 kcal/1050 kJ, 20 g carbohydrate, 5 g fibre, 26 g protein, 8 g fat

4 small chicken portions	*300 ml/½ pint skimmed milk*
1 green pepper, seeded and thinly sliced	*25 g/1 oz fine wholemeal flour*
	pinch of nutmeg
225 g/8 oz sweetcorn	*salt and pepper*
15 g/½ oz polyunsaturated margarine	*2 egg whites*
	25 g/1 oz wholemeal breadcrumbs

Heat the oven to 180°C/350°F/Gas 4. Lightly grease an ovenproof dish with oil. Grill the chicken briskly on all sides until brown. Place in the dish with the green pepper and corn.

Mix the margarine, cold milk and flour in a saucepan and bring to the boil, stirring constantly. Add the nutmeg, salt and pepper and cool a little.

Beat the egg whites until stiff but not dry and fold gently into the sauce. Pour over the chicken and sprinkle with the breadcrumbs. Bake in the oven for 40 minutes.

Serve with plain boiled brown rice and a salad.

Pollo con naranja   *Mexico*
*Chicken with orange

Serves 4

Each serving: 162 kcal/680 kJ, 10 g carbohydrate, 1 g fibre, 21 g protein, 4 g fat

4 chicken pieces	*pepper, to taste*
grated rind and juice of 3 oranges	*25 g/1 oz fine wholemeal flour*
200 ml/7 fl oz chicken stock (see page 29)	*4 tbsp water*
	2 tbsp smatana (see page 26)
	½ tsp cornflour

Grill the chicken pieces until golden on all sides. Put them into a saucepan with the orange rind, orange juice, chicken stock and pepper. Bring to the boil, cover and simmer for 30-40 minutes, or until the chicken is cooked and tender. Remove the chicken pieces to a heated serving dish and keep warm.

Mix the flour with the cold water and stir in a little of the cooking liquid. Add this to the saucepan and bring to the boil.

Mix the smatana with the cornflour and stir in a little of the liquid. Return to the pan and reheat. Pour the sauce over the chicken.

Serve with brown rice and a green vegetable.

MEAT

Dai suen chow yueng gone   *China*
***Liver stir-fried with leeks   See photograph, page 64

Serves 4 as part of a Chinese meal with other dishes

Each serving: 227 kcal/952 kJ, 15 g carbohydrate, 3 g fibre, 13 g protein, 13 g fat

225 g/8 oz *lamb's liver, cut into*
  5 mm × 5 cm/¼ × 2 in slices
2 tbsp cornflour
2 tbsp light soy sauce
1 tbsp dry sherry
300 ml/½ pint water

2 tbsp oil
225 g/8 oz *leeks, cut into 1 cm/½ in*
  slices
3 spring onions, sliced
1 tsp grated fresh ginger
50 g/2 oz mushrooms, sliced

Soak the liver in cold water for 15 minutes. Drain and dry.

Mix half the cornflour with half the soy sauce and the sherry and add the liver, coating it well with the mixture. Mix together the rest of the cornflour and the water and set aside.

Heat half the oil in a wok or non-stick frying pan and fry the liver quickly until it changes colour. Remove with a slotted spoon and drain on kitchen paper.

Put the remaining oil in the wok and add the leeks, spring onions, ginger and mushrooms and stir-fry over a high heat for 2-3 minutes. Return the liver to the wok with the remaining soy sauce and the cornflour and water mixture and bring to the boil. Simmer until it is thick.

Serve hot with plain boiled brown rice and one or two Chinese vegetable dishes, such as Choi nga choi or Ma tai chow hor lan dow (see page 91).

Badinghan mahshi bil-lahm
*Stuffed aubergines

Middle East

Serves 4

**Each serving: 191 kcal/801 kJ, 30 g carbohydrate, 7 g fibre,
13 g protein, 4 g fat**

2 large or 4 small aubergines
salt
85 g/3 oz yellow split peas
50 g/2 oz brown rice
1 tsp sunflower oil
1 small onion, finely chopped

100 g/3½ oz lean minced lamb
2 tbsp chopped fresh parsley
½ tsp ground cumin
½ tsp allspice
1 tbsp tomato purée
pepper, to taste

Split the aubergines lengthways and scoop out the pulp with a large spoon. Sprinkle with salt and set aside to drain in a colander for 30 minutes. Rinse off all the salt and finely chop the aubergine pulp.

Meanwhile, put the split peas and the rice into a saucepan with just enough water to cover. Bring to the boil, cover and simmer over a very low heat for 40-50 minutes until the rice and split peas are very soft. Drain off any surplus water.

Heat the oven to 200°C/400°F/Gas 6. Heat the oil in a non-stick pan and gently fry the onion until soft. Mix with the aubergine pulp and the rest of the ingredients. Cook for 2-3 minutes.

Fill the aubergine shells with the mixture and put into a baking dish with enough water to come halfway up the aubergines. Bake for 1 hour, or until the aubergines are soft.

Kibbeh bil sanieh
**Baked cracked wheat and lamb

Lebanon

Serves 4

**Each serving: 275 kcal/1153 kJ, 25 g carbohydrate, 2 g fibre,
20 g protein, 12 g fat**

Filling:
1 tsp oil
1 small onion
150 g/5 oz lean minced lamb
½ tsp allspice
15 g/½ oz pine nuts
25 g/1 oz raisins

Burghul mixture:
150 g/5 oz lean minced lamb
1 onion
½ tsp allspice
salt and pepper
100 g/3½ oz burghul (see page 25),
washed

7 g/¼ oz polyunsaturated margarine

Make the filling: heat the oil in a non-stick pan and fry the onion until it is soft. Add the minced meat and fry until brown. Stir in the allspice, pine nuts and raisins. Set aside to cool.

Put the meat, onion, allspice and salt and pepper into a food processor or blender and reduce to a paste. Alternatively, grind to a paste with a pestle and mortar. Add the burghul and continue to process or pound until it has become a smooth paste. It may be necessary to add a little water.

Heat the oven to 200°C/400°F/Gas 6. Lightly grease a 750 ml/1¼ pint shallow ovenproof dish. Spread half the burghul mixture on the bottom, cover with the filling and spread the other half of the burghul mixture over the top. Melt the margarine and brush it over the top. Mark the top into diamond shapes with a knife and run the knife around the sides of the dish. Bake in the oven for 40-50 minutes, until the top is browned.

Serve with a cucumber and yoghurt salad or any green vegetable.

Shish-kebab   *Middle East*
***Lamb kebabs

Serves 4

Each serving: 173 kcal/727 kJ, 5 g carbohydrate, 2 g fibre, 19 g protein, 9 g fat

Marinade:	Kebabs:
½ *small onion*	*8 pickling onions*
juice of 2 lemons	*8 small button mushrooms*
pepper, to taste	*1 tsp oil*
	8 very small tomatoes
340 g/12 oz lean lamb from the leg,	*1 green pepper, seeded and cut into*
cut into 2.5 cm/1 in cubes	*8 chunks*
	1 red pepper, seeded and cut into
	8 chunks

Make the marinade the day before serving the shish-kebab: purée the onion in a food processor or liquidizer with the lemon juice. Alternatively, crush it in a pestle and mortar and mix with the juice. Put into a bowl, season with the pepper and add the lamb. Cover and leave to marinate overnight in the refrigerator.

Parboil the onions for 3-4 minutes. Leave to cool. Blanch the mushrooms for 1 minute in boiling water, cool and brush with the oil.

When ready to cook the shish-kebab, thread the meat and vegetables alternately on to four long skewers and cook over charcoal or under a grill, basting with the marinade and turning the skewers from time to time, for 12-15 minutes, or until the meat is brown on the outside but still a little pink in the centre.

Serve on a bed of brown rice pilav with a green salad or Laban salateen (see page 107).

Yakní
Arab
*Vegetable and meat stew

Serves 4

Each serving: 209 kcal/880 kJ, 25 g carbohydrate, 8 g fibre, 18 g protein, 5 g fat

225 g/8 oz potatoes
1 tbsp sunflower oil
1 large onion, sliced
4 cloves garlic, crushed
½ tsp ground coriander
225 g/8 oz stewing veal, diced
115 g/4 oz okra, stems removed (see page 26)
1 courgette, sliced

1 small aubergine, cubed
115 g/4 oz green beans, sliced
225 g/8 oz spinach, chopped or 115 g/4 oz cabbage
3 tbsp tomato purée
3 tbsp chopped fresh parsley
½ tsp ground allspice
pepper, to taste
600 ml/1 pint water

Boil the potatoes, drain and cut into large chunks. Heat 2 teaspoons of the oil in a large non-stick frying pan and fry the onion, garlic and ground coriander until the onion is lightly browned. Add the meat and brown on all sides. Add the whole okra, courgette, aubergine, green beans and spinach or cabbage and gently fry until they also begin to brown. Add the tomato purée, parsley, allspice, pepper and the water. Bring to the boil, cover tightly and simmer for 1-1½ hours until the meat is tender and the sauce well reduced. Check occasionally and add more water if the stew is becoming dry.

In another non-stick pan, gently fry the potatoes in the remaining oil until they are brown. When the stew is ready for serving, stir in the potatoes and reheat.

Serve with plain boiled rice.

Note: If you wish, substitute 450 g/1 lb prepared weight of vegetables of your choice.

Chilli con carne
Mexico
*Red kidney beans with minced beef

Serves 4

Each serving: 220 kcal/925 kJ, 30 g carbohydrate, 16 g fibre, 19 g protein, 3 g fat

225 g/8 oz red kidney beans, soaked overnight
1 large onion, finely chopped
1 clove garlic, finely chopped
1 tsp sunflower oil
100 g/3½ oz lean minced beef

1 unseeded green chilli, finely chopped or ½-1 tsp dried chilli powder
1 bay leaf
1 × 400 g/14 oz can tomatoes with juice, chopped
salt and pepper

▶

Drain the beans, cover with fresh water and bring to the boil. Boil vigorously for 10 minutes, then lower the heat, cover and simmer for 1½-2 hours (30-45 minutes in a pressure cooker) until they are soft but still whole.

Fry the onion and garlic in the oil in a non-stick saucepan until soft. Add the meat and brown. Add the remainder of the ingredients and the cooked beans, cover and simmer for 45-60 minutes.

Serve with a green salad, brown rice or wholemeal bread.

Pastel de tamale   *Mexico*
*Minced beef pie with a cornmeal topping

Serves 4

Each serving: 262 kcal/1100 kJ, 30 g carbohydrate, 10 g fibre, 22 g protein, 7 g fat

1 large onion, chopped
1 tsp sunflower oil
225 g/8 oz lean minced beef
1 clove garlic
2 × 400 g/14 oz cans tomatoes, drained and chopped
225 g/8 oz shelled peas, fresh or frozen
1 tsp mild chilli powder

¼ tsp dried oregano
¼ tsp dried thyme
salt and pepper

Topping:
100 g/3½ oz cornmeal
1 egg
115 ml/4 fl oz skimmed milk
6 stuffed olives, halved

Brown the onion in the oil. Add the minced beef and cook until brown. Pour off any grease that has accumulated and add the garlic, tomatoes, peas, chilli, oregano, thyme, salt and pepper. Bring to the boil, lower the heat and simmer, uncovered, until the mixture is thick, about 10-15 minutes. Transfer the mixture to a lightly greased 1.5 l/2½ pint ovenproof dish. Heat the oven to 180°C/350°F/Gas 4.

Make the topping: mix the cornmeal, egg and milk together and pour the batter over the meat mixture. Garnish with the olives.

Bake for 30 minutes, or until set and lightly browned on top.

Serve with a green salad.

Picadillo
**Meat hash

Serves 5

**Each serving: 229 kcal/960 kJ, 20 g carbohydrate, 4 g fibre,
22 g protein, 7 g fat**

225 g/8 oz potatoes
1 tsp sunflower oil
225 g/8 oz lean minced beef
225 g/8 oz rabbit, minced
1 large onion, chopped
1 clove garlic, crushed
1 tbsp tomato purée
1 green chilli, seeded and finely
    chopped
225 g/8 oz cooking apples, peeled
    and chopped

225 g/8 oz canned tomatoes with
    juice
25 g/1 oz raisins
1 tsp dried oregano
2 cloves
25 g/1 oz stuffed olives
salt and pepper

Garnish:
15 g/½ oz flaked almonds, toasted

Boil the potatoes, drain and dice. Heat the oil in a non-stick saucepan and
brown the beef and rabbit together. Remove the meat with a slotted spoon
and set aside. Pour off any fat that has accumulated. Add the onion and
garlic and cook over a medium heat until brown. Return the meat to the
pan and add the tomato purée, chilli, apples, tomatoes, raisins, oregano
and cloves and bring to the boil. Cover and simmer for 20 minutes.

Add the potatoes and olives and simmer for a further 5 minutes. Season
to taste.

Serve sprinkled with the almonds, surrounded by brown rice, or with
tortillas.

Papas con chorizo
**Potatoes with sausage

Serves 4

**Each serving: 206 kcal/866 kJ, 25 g carbohydrate, 4 g fibre, 9 g protein,
8 g fat**

50 g/2 oz chorizo (see page 25),
    skinned and chopped
1 small onion, finely chopped
450 g/1 lb potatoes, cut into 5 mm/
    ¼ in dice

1 green pepper, seeded and finely
    chopped
3 tomatoes, sliced
50 g/2 oz low-fat Cheddar cheese,
    grated

Fry the chorizo in a non-stick frying pan until the fat begins to run. Add
the onion, potatoes and pepper, cover and fry gently for about 20-25
minutes, until the potatoes are soft. Cover with the sliced tomatoes,
sprinkle with the cheese, and brown under a grill until the cheese melts.

Serve with a green salad or green vegetables.

VEGETABLE MAIN DISHES

Ho yau dow fu   *China*
***Bean curd with oyster sauce

Serves 2 as a main dish with rice or 4 as part of an oriental meal

Each serving for 2: 185 kcal/775 kJ, 10 g carbohydrate, 2 g fibre, 8 g protein, 11 g fat
Each serving for 4: 92 kcal/388 kJ, 5 g carbohydrate, 1 g fibre, 4 g protein, 6 g fat

2 tsp cornflour
225 ml/8 fl oz water
2 tbsp oyster sauce
1 tbsp sunflower oil

285 g/10 oz black tofu (see page 26), cut into 14 × 5 mm/¹/₄ in pieces
100 g/3¹/₂ oz mushrooms, thinly sliced
4 spring onions, finely chopped

Mix together the cornflour, water and oyster sauce. Heat the sunflower oil in a non-stick frying pan and fry the tofu on both sides until light brown. Drain on absorbent paper.

Fry the mushrooms and most of the spring onions briefly – they should be hot but still crisp. Stir in the oyster sauce mixture and cook until it thickens. Return the tofu to the pan and reheat.

Serve with brown rice garnished with the remaining spring onions.

Note: Oyster sauce is a delicious flavouring. It is excellent with rice dishes and, surprisingly, stir-fried beef dishes.

If served as a main course with rice, precede this dish with a high protein soup such as Suk mai hai yuk tong (see page 30).

Mee goreng   *Malaysia*
*Fried noodles

Serves 4

Each serving: 404 kcal/1697 kJ, 70 g carbohydrate, 10 g fibre, 16 g protein, 8 g fat

340 g/12 oz wholewheat noodles or spaghetti
1 tbsp sunflower oil
285 g/10 oz black tofu (see page 26), cut into about 30 cubes
1 large onion, sliced

1 clove garlic, crushed
1 tbsp light soy sauce
2 tsp tomato purée
1 tsp chilli sauce
3 spring onions, sliced
170 g/6 oz potato, cooked and diced

Cook the noodles in boiling water for 3-5 minutes, or according to the package directions. Drain and rinse in cold water.

Heat 1 teaspoon of oil in a non-stick pan and fry the tofu until light brown. Drain on kitchen paper and set aside.

Add the rest of the oil to the pan and fry the onion and garlic until soft. Add the drained noodles, soy sauce, tomato purée, chilli sauce and the spring onions, reserving a little for a garnish. Toss over a medium heat for 1-2 minutes. Add the noodles and the tofu and stir-fry until everything is hot. Stir in the potatoes and heat through.

Serve garnished with the remaining spring onion accompanied by a crisp, fresh salad or Dhania raita (see page 41).

Khitchri
India

*Vegetable kedgeree

Serves 4

Each serving: 399 kcal/1676 kJ, 70 g carbohydrate, 14 g fibre, 19 g protein, 6 g fat

170 g/6 oz long-grain brown rice, washed
170 g/6 oz channa dhal (see page 25), or yellow split peas
600 ml/1 pint water
1 tbsp sunflower oil
2 tsp cumin seeds
1 tsp ground coriander
1/2 tsp turmeric

2 onions, chopped
1 small cauliflower, broken into florets
100 g/3 1/2 oz shelled peas, fresh or frozen
100 g/3 1/2 oz cut green beans
100 g/3 1/2 oz carrots, diced
2 tomatoes, skinned and chopped
1 tsp garam masala

Put the rice and split peas into a large saucepan with the water and bring to the boil. Then lower the heat, cover and simmer for 30-40 minutes, checking from time to time to ensure that the mixture has not boiled dry. Add more water if necessary. When cooked the rice and split peas should be tender but not mushy.

Meanwhile, heat the oil and fry the cumin seeds for a moment. Add the coriander and turmeric with the mixed vegetables, cover and fry gently for about 15 minutes, or until they are just cooked.

Stir the vegetables into the rice mixture with the garam masala.

Serve immediately with Dhania raita (see page 41) and Imli chatney (see page 40).

Sholay   *India*
**Quick chick pea curry

Serves 4

Each serving: 199 kcal/836 kJ, 30 g carbohydrate, 7 g fibre, 10 g protein, 6 g fat

1 large onion, sliced
15 g/½ oz polyunsaturated margarine
1-2 green chillies
4 cloves garlic, finely chopped
2.5 cm/1 in fresh ginger

150 ml/¼ pint water
1 tsp garam masala
1 tsp tomato purée
½ tsp curry powder
1 × 400 g/14 oz can chick peas

Fry the onion in the margarine in a non-stick pan until brown. Put the chillies, garlic, ginger and water into a food processor or blender and process until smooth. Add to the onion and cook for a few minutes, stirring. Add the garam masala, tomato purée, curry powder and chick peas, including the liquid from the can, and simmer gently for 15 minutes.

Serve with plain boiled brown rice and sliced tomatoes.

Uppama   *India*
**Semolina with vegetables

Serves 4

Each serving: 261 kcal/1097 kJ, 40 g carbohydrate, 7 g fibre, 10 g protein, 9 g fat

2 tbsp sunflower oil
2 tsp mustard seeds
1 dried red pepper
25 g/1 oz channa dhal (see page 25) or red lentils
1 large onion, finely chopped
1 green chilli
1 tsp grated fresh ginger
150 g/5 oz green cabbage, finely shredded

100 g/3½ oz potatoes cut into small dice
100 g/3½ oz shelled peas, fresh or frozen
115 g/4 oz wholewheat semolina
600 ml/1 pint boiling water

Garnish:
chopped fresh coriander or parsley

Heat the oil in a large non-stick frying pan and add the mustard seeds, red pepper and dhal. Fry gently for about 2-3 minutes shaking and stirring constantly. Add the onion, chilli, ginger, cabbage, potato and peas. Stir and fry for 2-3 minutes. Cover and simmer for about 5 minutes, or until the potatoes are just cooked. Add the semolina and cook gently for a further 5 minutes.

Add the water a little at a time, stirring gently, and allowing it to become absorbed between additions. Cook over a low heat for about 10 minutes, stirring occasionally until the grains swell.

Serve hot, garnished with coriander or parsley, with salad, chutney or pickle.

Mattar panir
***Peas with fresh cheese

India

Serves 4

Each serving: 260 kcal/1091 kJ, 15 g carbohydrate, 8 g fibre, 17 g protein, 16 g fat

2 cloves garlic
2.5 cm/1 in fresh ginger
1 green chilli
½ tsp turmeric
2 tsp ground coriander
2 tsp ground cumin
1 tbsp sunflower oil

225 g/8 oz ricotta cheese, cut into slices 1 cm/½ in thick
1 onion, chopped
1 × 400 g/14 oz can tomatoes, drained and chopped, liquid reserved
salt, to taste
340 g/12 oz shelled peas, fresh or frozen

Put the garlic, ginger, chilli, turmeric, coriander and cumin into a blender or food processor with just enough water to make a thick paste. Process until it is smooth. Alternatively, grind the ingredients in a pestle and mortar adding a little water when everything is crushed.

Heat the oil in a non-stick frying pan and fry the cheese until it is light brown on both sides. Drain on absorbent paper.

Fry the onion gently with the lid on the pan until it is soft. Add the spice paste and fry for about 4 minutes, or until the solids start to separate from the liquid. Add the tomatoes and cook for a further 5 minutes. Make up the tomato juice to 150 ml/¼ pint with water and add to the pan with a little salt to taste. Simmer gently with the lid on for 20 minutes. Add the peas and fried cheese and simmer for a further 7-10 minutes, until the peas are cooked.

Serve with brown rice or any wholemeal flatbread.

Koushari
*Lentil, macaroni and rice

Egypt

Serves 6

Each serving: 315 kcal/1324 kJ, 55 g carbohydrate, 8 g fibre, 13 g protein, 6 g fat

170 g/6 oz small brown lentils, washed
750 ml/1¼ pints plus 600 ml/1 pint water
100 g/3½ oz small wholewheat macaroni
salt, to taste
2 tbsp sunflower oil

170 g/6 oz brown Italian rice, washed and drained
450 g/1 lb onions, thinly sliced
2 cloves garlic, finely chopped
1 × 400 g/14 oz can tomatoes, chopped
2 tbsp tomato purée

Put the lentils and 750 ml/1¼ pints water into a saucepan, bring to the boil, then cover and simmer for about 1 hour until they are tender but still whole. Drain and set aside.

Boil the macaroni in plenty of lightly salted water for 15 minutes, or until soft but still firm. Set aside.

Heat half the oil in a saucepan and fry the rice for 1-2 minutes, add the 600 ml/1 pint water and a little salt. Bring to the boil, cover and simmer for 30-40 minutes, or until tender. Drain if necessary.

Heat the remaining oil in a pan and gently fry the onions and garlic until golden brown. Set aside.

Cook the tomatoes with their juice in an uncovered pan until they are well reduced and thick. Stir in the tomato purée.

Drain the macaroni and, using a fork, mix lightly into the rice with the lentils. Add half the onion mixture and all the tomato sauce. Reheat. Transfer to a serving dish and garnish with the rest of the onions.

Serve with a crisp green salad.

Rishla peynirli yoghurt salsai   *Middle East*
**Noodles with yoghurt cheese sauce

Serves 4

**Each serving: 378 kcal/1589 kJ, 50 g carbohydrate, 6 g fibre,
23 g protein, 11 g fat**

Cheese sauce:
15 g/½ oz polyunsaturated
  margarine
25 g/1 oz fine wholemeal flour
450 ml/¾ pint low-fat plain yoghurt
  (see page 45)
100 g/3½ oz low-fat Cheddar
  cheese, grated

½ tsp allspice
1 tsp paprika
salt and pepper

225 g/8 oz wholewheat noodles

To serve:
25 g/1 oz Parmesan cheese, grated

Make the sauce: put the margarine, flour and yoghurt into a saucepan. Bring to the boil over a medium heat, whisking vigorously with a sauce whisk until it thickens. Remove from the heat and add the cheese and the spices and seasoning. Set aside.

Cook the noodles according to the packet directions. Drain. Reheat the cheese sauce and mix in the drained noodles.

Serve with a generous sprinkling of Parmesan cheese accompanied by green salad.

Turlu   *Turkey*
*Mixed vegetable stew

Serves 4

**Each serving: 147 kcal/617 kJ, 20 g carbohydrate, 11 g fibre,
8 g protein, 4 g fat**

100 g/3½ oz haricot beans, soaked
  overnight
1 tbsp olive oil

1 onion, chopped
2 cloves garlic, finely chopped
1 carrot, peeled and sliced

225 g/8 oz French beans, topped
   and tailed
1 × 400 g/14 oz can tomatoes
225 g/8 oz courgettes, sliced

2 tbsp tomato purée
salt and pepper

Garnish:
   chopped fresh parsley

Drain the beans, cover with fresh water and bring to the boil. Boil vigorously for 10 minutes, then lower the heat, cover and simmer for 1-1½ hours or omit the soaking and cook the beans for 25-30 minutes in a pressure cooker. Drain and set aside, reserving the liquid.

Heat the oil in a large saucepan and gently fry the onion until it begins to brown. Add the rest of the ingredients. Cover and simmer gently for 30-45 minutes, until the vegetables are very well cooked. Add salt and pepper to taste.

Sprinkle with parsley and serve hot or at room temperature with pitta bread or a plain pilav.

Note: Use any vegetables of your choice as substitutes for those suggested in this recipe.

Bulgur pilavi
Middle East
*Burghul pilav with aubergines and cheese

Serves 4

Each serving: 292 kcal/1227 kJ, 50 g carbohydrate, 6 g fibre, 15 g protein, 6 g fat

2 aubergines, cubed
salt
1 tsp sunflower oil
1 onion, finely chopped
225 g/8 oz burghul (cracked wheat,
   see page 25), washed

400 ml/14 fl oz water
100 g/3½ oz low-fat Cheddar
   cheese, cut into tiny cubes
pepper, to taste

Put the aubergines in a colander, sprinkle with salt and allow to drain for 30 minutes. Rinse off the salt and dry with kitchen paper.

Heat the oil in a non-stick frying pan, add the onion, cover and fry gently for 5-10 minutes, until it is beginning to brown. Add the aubergines, cover and fry gently for 5 minutes. Add the burghul and fry gently for 1-2 minutes, tossing with a wooden fork to make sure the grains are coated with the oil. Add the water and a little salt and bring to the boil. Cover and simmer very slowly for 7-10 minutes, until all the water is absorbed. Turn off the heat. Put two layers of kitchen paper between the pan and the lid and leave to rest for 10 minutes.

Mix in the cheese and serve immediately, sprinkled liberally with pepper.

Ful medames
Simmered ful beans

Egypt

Serves 4

**Each serving with egg: 390 kcal/1634 kJ, 40 g carbohydrate, 15 g fibre, 25 g protein, 14 g fat*
Each serving without egg: 316 kcal/1325 kJ, 40 g carbohydrate, 15 g fibre, 19 g protein, 8 g fat

285 g/10 oz ful (see page 26), fava or small dried broad beans, soaked overnight
3 cloves garlic, crushed
1 tsp ground cumin

salt and pepper
4 hard-boiled eggs (optional)
2 tbsp olive oil
2 tbsp chopped fresh parsley
1 lemon, cut into wedges

Drain the beans, cover with fresh water and bring to the boil. Lower the heat, then cover and simmer for 4-6 hours (35-45 minutes in a pressure cooker) until they soft. Drain and add the garlic, cumin, salt and pepper.

Ladle into four bowls, top each with a hard-boiled egg, if using, dribble over a little olive oil and sprinkle with parsley.

Serve with lemon wedges and a tomato salad. As you eat it, squeeze the lemon juice over and mash the egg into the beans. This dish is also delicious served with soft-boiled eggs, the yolks forming a sauce for the beans.

Chiles rellenos con queso
***Peppers stuffed with cheese

Mexico

Serves 4

Each serving: 198 kcal/834 kJ, 15 g carbohydrate, 4 g fibre, 14 g protein, 9 g fat

Sauce:
1 onion, finely chopped
1 clove garlic, crushed
1 green chilli, finely chopped
1 tsp sunflower oil
1 × 400 g/14 oz can tomatoes, chopped
pepper, to taste
pinch of dried oregano

4 green peppers
100 g/3½ oz low-fat Cheddar cheese
2 egg whites
50 g/2 oz wholemeal flour
4 tbsp skimmed milk
1 tbsp sunflower oil

Make the sauce: gently fry the onion, garlic and chilli in the oil until golden. Add the tomatoes with their juice, pepper and oregano. Bring to the boil and simmer uncovered for about 15 minutes, until the sauce has thickened a little.

Meanwhile, grill the green peppers until they are brown on all sides. Put them into a plastic bag for 10-15 minutes. Take them out one at a time and pull the skin off gently. Remove the cores and seeds. Cut the cheese to fit inside the peppers and secure the tops with tooth picks.

Heat the oven to 200°C/400°F/Gas 6. Whisk the egg whites until they form soft peaks. Mix the flour with the milk and fold into the egg whites.

Heat the oil in a non-stick pan. Dip the peppers one at a time into the egg mixture. Place on a wet saucer and slide into the hot oil. Cook until golden brown and turn gently. Cook the other side. Transfer to a baking dish and pour over the tomato sauce. Bake for 10-15 minutes.

Serve with brown rice and a green salad.

Flan de legumbres
Ecuador
*Mixed vegetable bake

Serves 4

Each serving: 209 kcal/878 kJ, 25 g carbohydrate, 7 g fibre, 14 g protein, 6 g fat

400 g/14 oz frozen or fresh mixed vegetables
45 g/1½ oz lean bacon
3 eggs
300 ml/½ pint skimmed milk

100 g/3½ oz fresh wholemeal breadcrumbs
1 tbsp chopped fresh parsley
salt and pepper

Defrost the frozen vegetables or peel, dice and blanch fresh ones for 2-3 minutes in boiling water. Cool in cold water.

Heat the oven to 180°C/350°F/Gas 4. Grill the bacon until crisp, drain on kitchen paper and chop. Beat the eggs and milk together. Mix in the breadcrumbs, parsley, vegetables and bacon and season with salt and pepper. Pour into a lightly greased 900 ml/1½ pint, shallow ovenproof dish. Stand the dish in a roasting tin with hot water to come halfway up the dish and bake for 45-60 minutes or until a knife, inserted in the centre, comes out clean.

Frijoles refritos
Refried beans

Mexico

Serves 4-6, depending on how used

*Each serving for 4: 151 kcal/633 kJ, 25 g carbohydrate, 12 g fibre, 13 g protein, 2 g fat
*Each serving for 6: 100 kcal/422 kJ, 15 g carbohydrate, 8 g fibre, 8 g protein, 1 g fat

45 g/1½ oz lean bacon, diced
l large onion, chopped
1 clove garlic, chopped

500 g/17½ oz cooked pinto or red kidney beans, (175 g/6 oz bodyweight) or 2 × 400 g/14 oz can, drained with a little liquid reserved
salt and pepper

Fry the bacon in a non-stick pan until crisp. Drain on kitchen paper. Fry the onion and garlic in the remaining fat until brown.

Mash all but 2 tablespoons of the beans. Alternatively, work in a food processor with enough bean liquid to make a thick paste. Return the mashed and unmashed beans to the pan and reheat, adding salt and pepper to taste.

Eat with salad and bread or use to stuff tacos or vegetables. This quantity is enough to stuff 6 tacos or 6 peppers.

Ensalada de garbanzos
**Chick pea salad

Latin America

Serves 4

Each serving: 135 kcal/569 kJ, 15 g carbohydrate, 5 g fibre, 7 g protein, 6 g fat

225 g/8 oz cooked chick peas, (100 g/3½ oz dry weight), or 1 × 400 g/14 oz can, drained, with 2 tbsp liquid reserved
1 tbsp sunflower oil
1 tbsp lemon juice
2 tbsp tomato purée

1 tsp Dijon mustard
1 clove garlic, crushed
½ tsp mild chilli powder
2 tbsp chopped fresh parsley
2 spring onions, finely sliced
2 stalks celery, chopped
1 canned pimiento, drained and sliced

If using dried chick peas, drain them and cover with fresh water. Bring to the boil and boil for 10 minutes, lower the heat and simmer covered for about 1½ hours (30-40 minutes in a pressure cooker).

Mix together the oil, lemon juice, tomato purée, liquid from the chick peas, mustard, garlic, chilli powder and parsley. Stir in the remaining ingredients, reserving a few green onion tops and pimiento slices for garnish. Leave for 2-3 hours for the flavours to mingle.

Serve at room temperature, garnished with the reserved onion and pimiento as a starter or light meal.

ACCOMPANYING VEGETABLES AND SALADS

HOT DISHES

Ma tai chow hor lan dow *China*
**Stir-fried mange tout and water chestnuts

Serves 4 as part of an oriental meal   **See photograph, page 97**

Each serving: 125 kcal/527 kJ, 20 g carbohydrate, 1 g fibre, 3 g protein, 5 g fat

2 tsp cornflour	*1 × 230 g/8 oz can water chestnuts,*
4 tbsp dry sherry	*sliced*
1 tbsp sunflower oil	*170 ml/6 fl oz vegetable stock*
170 g/6 oz mange tout, topped and	*1 tbsp light soy sauce*
tailed	*1 tsp sesame oil*

Mix the cornflour with the sherry and set aside.

Heat the sunflower oil in a wok or a large non-stick pan and stir-fry the mange tout for about 3 minutes until lightly cooked but still crisp. Add the water chestnuts and the stock and simmer for 1-2 minutes. Stir in the sherry mixture and the soy sauce. Bring to the boil and simmer for 1 minute.

Sprinkle over the sesame oil and serve piping hot.

Choi nga choi *China*
***Stir-fried beansprouts

Serves 4   **See photograph, page 97**

Each serving: 58 kcal/242 kJ, negligible carbohydrate, 3 g fibre, 1 g protein, 5 g fat

1 tbsp sunflower oil	*300 g/10½ oz beansprouts*
1 tsp grated fresh ginger	*6 radishes, thinly sliced*
2 spring onions, cut the length of	*1 tbsp light soy sauce*
the beansprouts	*1 tsp sesame oil*

Heat the oil in a wok or non-stick frying pan and fry the ginger for a moment or two. Add the spring onions, beansprouts and radishes and stir-fry over a high heat for 1-2 minutes. Add the soy sauce and the sesame oil and serve immediately.

Aruna's aloo   *India*
*Aruna's potatoes with sauce

Serves 4

Each serving: 181 kcal/760 kJ, 30 g carbohydrate, 4 g fibre, 5 g protein, 5 g fat

450 g/1 lb potatoes, peeled and
 chopped
1 tbsp sunflower oil
1 tsp mustard seeds
1 large Spanish onion, finely
 chopped
1 × 200 g/7 oz can tomatoes,
 chopped
½ tsp turmeric

1 tsp chilli powder or to taste
2 cloves garlic, crushed
1 tsp grated fresh ginger
salt, to taste
2 tsp tomato purée
juice of ½ lemon
1 tsp garam masala
225 ml/8 fl oz water

Boil the potatoes in their skins, peel them and cut into large chunks. Heat the oil in a non-stick saucepan. Put in the mustard seeds and fry until they pop. Add the onion and cook gently, covered, until soft. Add the tomatoes, turmeric, chilli, garlic, ginger, salt and tomato purée and cook, covered, for 20 minutes, until the sauce is thick. Add the potatoes, lemon juice, garam masala and water and cook with the lid half on for about 15-20 minutes, until most of the water has evaporated and the sauce is thick.

Serve with Dhania raita (see page 41) or chutney.

Avtar's gobi sabji   *India*
*Punjabi cauliflower and potatoes

Serves 4

Each serving: 179 kcal/752 kJ, 30 g carbohydrate, 8 g fibre, 8 g protein, 4 g fat

15 g/½ oz polyunsaturated
 margarine
225 g/8 oz onions, finely chopped
2 tsp grated fresh ginger
1 green chilli, finely chopped
3 cloves garlic, finely chopped
2 tsp turmeric
1 tsp ground coriander
1 × 200 g/7 oz can tomatoes

1 × 900 g/2 lb cauliflower, broken
 into florets
340 g/12 oz potatoes, cut into
 2.5 cm/1 in cubes
salt, to taste
2-3 tbsp water
2 tsp garam masala
2 tbsp chopped fresh coriander

Heat the margarine in a large non-stick pan and fry the onions gently until soft. Add the ginger, chilli, garlic, turmeric and ground coriander. Fry for 3-4 minutes and stir in the tomatoes. Add the cauliflower florets and the leaves cut into small slices, the potatoes, a little salt and about 2 tablespoons of water. Bring to the boil, cover and simmer gently for 15-20 minutes, or until the vegetables are tender. Stir every few minutes and add a little more water if the mixture begins to stick.

Add the garam masala and coriander and serve hot with chapatis (see page 115).

Ravi's bean mallung
***French beans

Sri Lanka

Serves 4

Each serving: 69 kcal/292 kJ, 5 g carbohydrate, 2 g fibre, 2 g protein, 5 g fat

1 tbsp sunflower oil
1 large onion, thinly sliced
1 tbsp mustard seeds

225 g/8 oz French beans, fresh or frozen, topped and tailed, and halved

Heat the oil in a wok or frying pan and fry the onion until very brown. Add the mustard seeds and fry them until they begin to pop. Add the beans and stir-fry for about 5-7 minutes, or until they are cooked.

Afelia
***Mushrooms with coriander

Turkey

Serves 4

Each serving: 69 kcal/290 kJ, negligible carbohydrate, 3 g fibre, 2 g protein, 5 g fat

1 tbsp sunflower oil
1 tsp coriander seeds
450 g/1 lb mushrooms, quartered if large

115 ml/4 fl oz red wine
pepper, to taste

Heat the oil in a non-stick frying pan and fry the coriander seeds for a few moments. Add the mushrooms and fry lightly on both sides. Add the wine and a little pepper. Bring to the boil, cover, lower the heat and simmer for 10 minutes. Serve hot or at room temperature.

Coubish   *Middle East*
**Cabbage

Serves 4

Each serving: 90 kcal/377 kJ, 5 g carbohydrate, 5 g fibre, 6 g protein, 4 g fat

1 tsp coriander seeds	1 small cabbage, finely shredded
1 tbsp olive oil	salt and pepper
1 small onion	
2 tbsp tomato purée	
4 tbsp water	

Roast the coriander seeds in an ungreased heavy-based frying pan until they begin to brown.

Heat the oil in a large saucepan and fry the onion until soft. Stir in the tomato purée, coriander and water. Add the cabbage and season to taste. Cover tightly and cook over a low heat, stirring occasionally, for 5-10 minutes, or until the cabbage is just cooked.

Fasulye pilaki   *Turkey*
*Haricot bean stew

Serves 4

Each serving: 168 kcal/707 kJ, 25 g carbohydrate, 11 g fibre, 10 g protein, 4 g fat

170 g/6 oz haricot beans, soaked overnight	4 tbsp tomato purée
1 tbsp olive oil	¼ tsp mild chilli powder
1 onion, chopped	½ tsp allspice
1 clove garlic, finely chopped	juice of ½ lemon

Drain the beans, cover with fresh water and bring to the boil. Boil vigorously for 10 minutes, then lower the heat, cover and simmer for 1-1½ hours (25-30 minutes in a pressure cooker). Drain and set aside, reserving the liquid.

Heat the oil and fry the onion and garlic until soft. Add the beans with the tomato purée, chilli powder, allspice and 150 ml/¼ pint bean liquid. Bring to the boil, cover and lower the heat. Simmer over a very low heat for 30 minutes, adding more liquid halfway through, if necessary. The consistency of the completed dish should be similar to baked beans. If there is too much liquid, increase the heat and cook without the lid until you have the right amount; if it is too dry add a little more cooking liquid. Add the lemon juice and serve hot or at room temperature.

Havuc
**Carrots with coriander

Serves 4

Each serving: 39 kcal/165 kJ, 5 g carbohydrate, 3 g fibre, 1 g protein, 1 g fat

450 g/1 lb carrots, sliced
1 tsp sunflower oil
1 tsp ground coriander
juice of ½ lemon
salt and pepper

4 tbsp water

Garnish:
chopped fresh coriander or parsley

Gently fry the carrots in the oil in a non-stick saucepan until golden. Add the rest of the ingredients. Bring to the boil, cover and simmer for 10-15 minutes, or until cooked but still a little crisp. Garnish with the fresh coriander or parsley.

Kousah
***Purée of courgettes

Serves 4

Each serving: 64 kcal/270 kJ, 5 g carbohydrate, 3 g fibre, 1 g protein, 4 g fat

450 g/1 lb courgettes, thickly
   sliced
½ tsp salt
1 tbsp olive oil
1 small onion, finely chopped
225 g/8 oz tomatoes, skinned and
   chopped or 1 × 200 g/7 oz can,
   drained

juice of ½ lemon
freshly milled black pepper

Garnish:
1 tbsp chopped fresh parsley

Put the courgettes into a colander, sprinkle with the salt and set aside for 30 minutes to drain. Rinse and drain again.
   Heat the oil in a non-stick saucepan and add the onion. Cover and fry gently for 5-10 minutes until soft. Add the courgettes and fry for a further 5 minutes. Add the rest of the ingredients, cover and simmer gently for about 20 minutes, until the courgettes are soft. Purée in a food processor or liquidizer or mash well. Sprinkle with parsley and serve hot or cold.

Sabanikh mahshi bil-batata
Middle East

*Potatoes stuffed with spinach
See photograph, page 99

Serves 4

Each serving: 126 kcal/530 kJ, 25 g carbohydrate, 4 g fibre, 4 g protein, 1 g fat

2 × 225 g/8 oz potatoes, unpeeled
1 tsp sunflower oil
1 small onion
115 g/4 oz spinach, cooked, well
  drained and chopped
¼ tsp allspice
salt and pepper

Sauce:
2 tbsp tomato purée
150 ml/¼ pint water
pepper, to taste

Boil the potatoes in their skins until they are just cooked. Cut into halves lengthways and scoop out the centres, mash and set aside.

Heat the oil in a non-stick saucepan and gently fry the onion until soft. Add the spinach and allspice and season with salt and pepper. Add the mashed potato and pile into the shells. Put the potatoes in an oven-to-table dish, just large enough to hold them in one layer. Heat the oven to 200°C/400°F/Gas 6.

Make the sauce: mix the tomato purée with the water, season with pepper and bring to the boil. Pour the sauce over the potatoes and bake for 20-30 minutes.

Zeytinyagli pirasa
Turkey

**Braised leeks

Serves 4

Each serving: 86 kcal/360 kJ, 10 g carbohydrate, 5 g fibre, 4 g protein, 4 g fat

1 tbsp olive oil
1 small onion, finely chopped
4 tbsp tomato purée
115 ml/4 fl oz water
4 tbsp chopped fresh parsley

salt and pepper
juice of ½ lemon
450 g/1 lb leeks, halved
  lengthways

Choi nga choi (*above*, see page 91); Ma tai chow hor lan dow (*below*, see page 91).
OVERLEAF: Bamiah (*left*, see page 101); Sabanikh mahshi bil-batata (*top right*); Imam bayildi (*below right*, see page 101).

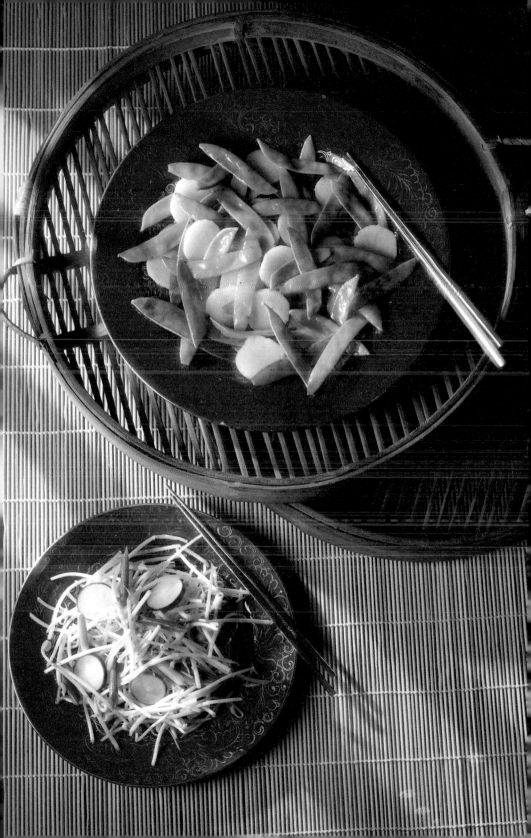

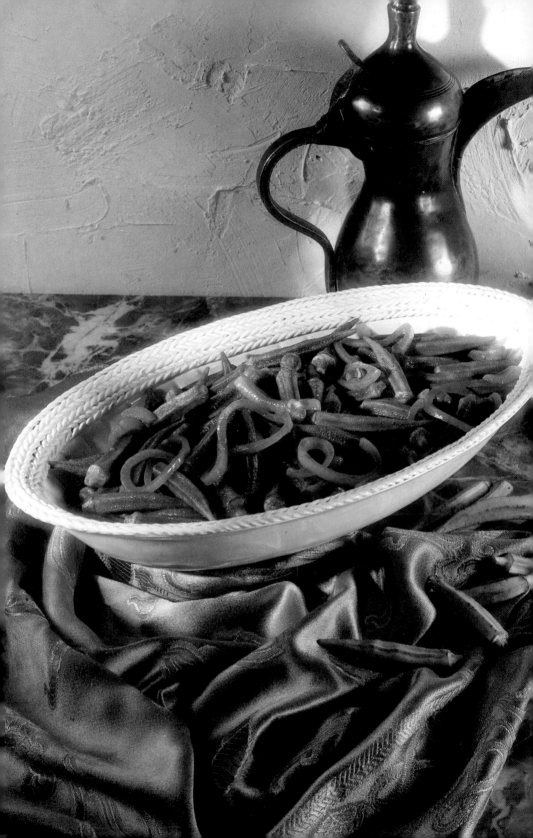

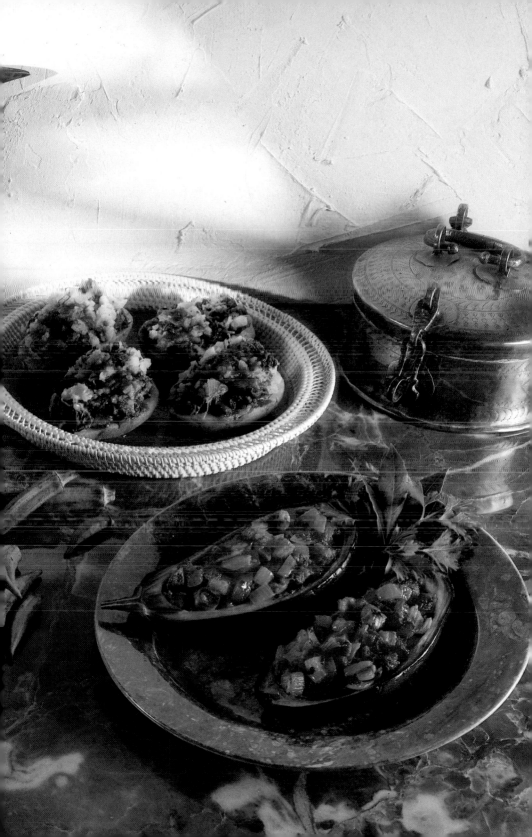

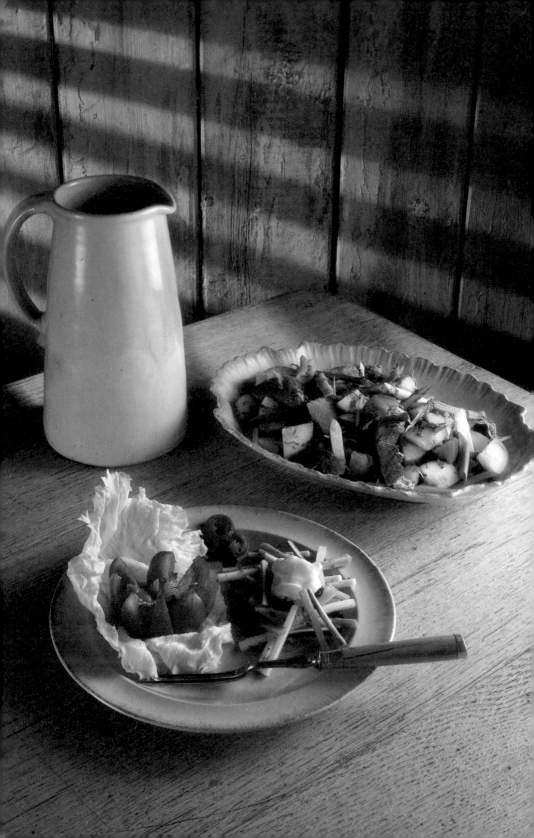

In a pan just large enough to take the leeks, heat the oil and gently fry the onion until it is soft. Add the tomato purée, water, half the parsley, the salt and pepper and the lemon juice. Bring to the boil. Add the leeks, cover and simmer over a low heat for 15-20 minutes. Transfer to a serving dish and sprinkle with the rest of the parsley. Serve hot or at room temperature.

Bamiah   *Middle East*
**Okra   See photograph, page 98

Serves 4

Each serving: 47 kcal/196 kJ, 5 g carbohydrate, 4 g fibre, 3 g protein, 1 g fat

1 tsp olive oil	*115 ml/4 fl oz water*
1 onion, sliced	*½ tsp turmeric*
450 g/1 lb okra (see page 26), stems	*½ tsp ground coriander*
removed	*salt and pepper*
2 tbsp tomato purée	*juice of 1 lemon*

Heat the oil in a non-stick pan and fry the onion over a low heat with the lid on until brown. Add the okra, tomato purée, water, spices and seasonings. Bring to the boil, cover, lower heat and simmer 30 minutes. Add the lemon juice and continue to simmer for a further 10 minutes.

Imam bayildi   *Turkey*
**Stuffed aubergines   See photograph, page 99

Serves 4

Each serving: 175 kcal/737 kJ, 20 g carbohydrate, 12 g fibre, 4 g protein, 9 g fat

4 aubergines, halved lengthways	*340 g/12 oz tomatoes, skinned and*
2 tsp salt	*chopped or 1 × 400 g/14 oz can,*
1 tsp plus 2 tbsp olive oil	*drained*
225 g/8 oz onions, finely chopped	*25 g/1 oz sultanas*
2 cloves garlic	*pepper, to taste*
1 tbsp chopped parsley	*1 bay leaf*
1 tsp chopped fresh thyme, or	*600 ml/1 pint water*
¼ tsp dried	

Hollow out the aubergine halves leaving a shell 1 cm/⅔ in thick. Reserve the aubergine flesh. Sprinkle the shells with the salt and invert for 30 minutes to drain off the excess liquid. Rinse off the salt and drain again.

Meanwhile, heat the oven to 150°C/350°F/Gas 2. Heat the teaspoon of oil in a non-stick pan and gently fry the onions and garlic until soft. Add the parsley, thyme, tomatoes, sultanas, reserved chopped aubergine flesh, pepper to taste and the bay leaf. Simmer uncovered, stirring occasionally for 10-15 minutes, or until thick. Discard the bay leaf.

Fattoush (*above*, see page 108); Jitomates rellenos (*below*, see page 109).

Spoon the mixture into the aubergine halves. Arrange in a baking dish, just large enough to hold all the aubergines in one layer. Pour in the water, and spoon the remaining oil over the aubergines. Bake in the oven for 1½-2 hours, until the aubergines are very soft. Discard the cooking liquid. Serve hot or cold.

Note: This dish is translated 'the fainting priest'. Legend has it that the Imam fainted because his new young wife had used too much expensive olive oil in its preparation. There will be no such problem with this oil-reduced version.

Coliflor con salsa de elote   *Mexico*
*Cauliflower with sweetcorn sauce

Serves 4

Each serving: 91 kcal/381 kJ, 15 g carbohydrate, 7 g fibre, 6 g protein, negligible fat

1 small cauliflower	*200 ml/⅓ pint skimmed milk*
225 g/8 oz fresh or frozen	*1 tsp paprika*
sweetcorn	*salt and pepper*
1 tbsp cornmeal	*cayenne pepper, to sprinkle*

Cook the cauliflower whole for 15-20 minutes, until tender. Cook the corn until soft. Put the corn, cornmeal, milk, paprika, salt and pepper into a food processor or blender and process until smooth.

Put the corn mixture into a saucepan and bring to the boil, stirring all the time. Simmer, still stirring until it is the consistency of a reasonably thick white sauce. Season and pour over the cauliflower. Garnish with a sprinkling of cayenne pepper.

Elote   *Mexico*
*Mexican corn

Serves 4

Each serving: 104 kcal/435 kJ, 20 g carbohydrate, 7 g fibre, 4 g protein, 2 g fat

1 tsp sunflower oil	*400 g/14 oz fresh or frozen*
1 small green pepper, seeded and	*sweetcorn*
finely chopped	*1 × 400 g/14 oz can tomatoes,*
1 small red pepper, seeded and finely	*drained and chopped*
chopped	*pepper, to taste*

Heat the oil in a non-stick saucepan. Add the peppers, cover and fry gently over a medium heat until they begin to turn colour. Add the corn, tomatoes and pepper and bring to the boil. Cover and simmer for 5-10 minutes, until the corn is tender. Serve hot.

Habas verdes y chiles
**Broad beans with peppers

Mexico

Serves 4

Each serving: 103 kcal/431 kJ, 15 g carbohydrate, 3 g fibre, 6 g protein, 3 g fat

*275 g/9½ oz shelled broad beans,
  fresh or frozen
2 tsp sunflower oil*

*1 small onion, finely chopped
½ green pepper, seeded and sliced
½ red pepper, seeded and sliced*

Cook the beans for 10-15 minutes, or until just soft. Meanwhile, heat the oil in a non-stick saucepan and fry the onion gently with the lid on until soft. Add the peppers, cover again and fry gently for 10-15 minutes, or until they have softened and lost their bright colours.

Drain the beans and mix with the peppers.

Calabacitas con chiles rojas
**Courgettes with sweet red peppers

Mexico

Serves 4

Each serving: 59 kcal/249 kJ, 5 g carbohydrate, 3 g fibre, 2 g protein, 3 g fat

*1 small onion, chopped
2 tsp sunflower oil
450 g/1 lb small courgettes, sliced
salt and pepper*

*1 × 200 g/7 oz can red pimientos
4 tbsp smatana (see page 26)
  or Greek yoghurt*

Fry the onion gently in the oil in a covered non-stick pan until soft. Add the courgettes, and a little salt and pepper. Cover and continue to cook slowly for 10-15 minutes until just soft, shaking the pan from time to time.

Purée the pimientos in a food processor or blender. Alternatively, mince or chop very finely. Add to the courgettes. Reheat, remove from the heat and stir in the smatana.

Ejotes con jugo de lima
***Green beans in lime juice

Mexico

Serves 4

Each serving: 37 kcal/155 kJ, negligible carbohydrate, 4 g fibre, 1 g protein, 3 g fat

*450 g/1 lb French beans, fresh or
  frozen, topped and tailed and
  halved*

*15 g/½ oz polyunsaturated
  margarine
1 tbsp chopped fresh parsley
pepper, to taste
juice of 1 lime*

Cook the beans in the minimum quantity of boiling water until just tender. Drain well.

Melt the margarine in a large non-stick frying pan. Add the beans and fry gently until they begin to lose their bright green colour. Add the parsley, pepper and lime juice and serve immediately.

Calabacitas con elote   *Mexico*
**Courgettes with corn

Serves 4

Each serving: 118 kcal/496 kJ, 20 g carbohydrate, 5 g fibre, 3 g protein, 4 g fat

15 g/½ oz polyunsaturated   *salt and pepper*
  margarine
1 small onion, chopped   *Garnish:*
450 g/1 lb courgettes, diced   *chopped fresh parsley*
225 g/8 oz sweetcorn kernels

Heat the margarine in a non-stick frying pan and fry the onion with the lid on until soft. Add the courgettes, corn, salt and pepper. Cover and fry gently for 5-7 minutes, shaking the pan frequently, or until the courgettes are cooked but still a little crisp. Garnish with chopped parsley.

Serve hot. This dish is delicious as an accompaniment to fish.

SALADS

Tim suen yeh choi sa lud
China

*Sweet and sour cabbage salad

Serves 4

Each serving: 65 kcal/274 kJ, 10 g carbohydrate, 5 g fibre, 4 g protein, 1 g fat

*450 g/1 lb white cabbage, cored
   and leaves separated
1 tsp sunflower oil
1 red pepper, seeded, cored and
   finely chopped*

*2 tbsp light soy sauce
2 tbsp unsweetened apple
   concentrate
2 tbsp wine vinegar*

Plunge the cabbage leaves into a large pan of boiling water. Boil for 3-4 minutes, until they are just tender. Drain and cool. Starting at the stalk end, roll the leaves, Swiss-roll style. Cut them into 2½ cm/1 in slices and arrange decoratively on a serving plate.

Heat the oil in a non-stick pan and fry the pepper for 1-2 minutes. Add the soy sauce, apple concentrate and vinegar. Bring to the boil and pour over the cabbage. Serve chilled.

Goma-ae
Japan

***Broccoli and mooli salad

Serves 4

Each serving: 92 kcal/388 kJ, 5 g carbohydrate, 3 g fibre, 5 g protein, 6 g fat

*225 g/8 oz broccoli, divided into
   small florets
225 g/8 oz mooli (see page 26),
   peeled and coarsely grated*

*3 tbsp sesame seeds
1 tbsp shoyu or light soy sauce
3 tbsp water*

Drop the broccoli florets into boiling water for 1 minute, then into cold water to cool them quickly. Drain thoroughly.

Arrange the mooli on a flat serving dish or four individual bowls and mound the broccoli in the centre. Chill until ready to serve.

Heat the sesame seeds in a heavy-based ungreased frying pan. Fry until they begin to jump. Grind to a powder in a coffee grinder or with a pestle and mortar. Mix in the shoyu and water. Pour over the salad when ready to serve.

Ohhitashi
***Spinach salad with sesame seed dressing

Japan

Serves 4

Each serving: 76 kcal/321 kJ, 5 g carbohydrate, 5 g fibre, 5 g protein, 4 g fat

450 g/1 lb fresh spinach
2 tbsp sesame seeds

2 tbsp shoyu or light soy sauce
2 tbsp water

Wash and drain the spinach. Divide it into two piles, stems together and leaves together. Tie each bunch firmly with string at 5 cm/2 in intervals so that the spinach forms two long rolls. Plunge them into a large pan of boiling water, bring to a vigorous boil and cook for 3 minutes. Drain and plunge into cold water. Drain again and squeeze out all the liquid using a bamboo sushi mat or a clean tea-towel, making the spinach into long, tight rolls. Cool.

Remove the string and cut each spinach roll into 4 cm/1½ in slices.

While the spinach is cooling, toast the sesame seeds in an heavy-based ungreased frying pan until they begin to pop. Set aside 1 teaspoon for garnish and grind the rest in a coffee grinder or with a pestle and mortar. Mix with the shoyu, or soy sauce, and water and pour on to a serving platter large enough to take all the spinach. Arrange the spinach rolls attractively over the dressing and sprinkle with the reserved sesame seeds.

Note: For a quicker method, simply blanch the washed spinach for 1 minute in boiling water. Drain well, chop coarsely and divide it between four bowls. Pour a little dressing over each portion.

Gajar aney rai
***Gujerati carrot salad

India

Serves 4

Each serving: 64 kcal/270 kJ, 5 g carbohydrate, 3 g fibre, 1 g protein, 4 g fat

340 g/12 oz carrots, grated
1 tbsp sunflower oil
1 tsp mustard seeds

1 tsp fenugreek seeds (optional)
pepper, to taste

Put the carrots into a salad bowl. Heat the oil in a small saucepan and fry the mustard seeds and the fenugreek seeds, if using, until they pop. Pour over the carrots and stir in with pepper, to taste.

Pyaaz sambal
*Onion salad

India

Serves 4

Each serving: 26 kcal/108 kJ, 5 g carbohydrate, 3 g fibre, 1 g protein, negligible fat

a few lettuce leaves
1 lemon
1 large Spanish onion, very finely sliced

1 green chilli, seeded and finely chopped

Line a flat dish with the lettuce leaves. Cut half the lemon into thin slices and arrange with the onion slices on the lettuce. Squeeze the other half of the lemon and sprinkle the juice over the salad. Garnish with the chilli. Serve with tandoori dishes or curry.

Salatah al-adas
*Lentil salad

Middle East

Serves 4

Each serving: 221 kcal/930 kJ, 35 g carbohydrate, 7 g fibre, 14 g protein, 4 g fat

1 tbsp sunflower oil
1 onion, chopped
2 cloves garlic, finely chopped
225 g/8 oz green lentils, washed and drained

½ tsp ground cumin
½ tsp ground coriander
600 ml/1 pint water
juice and grated rind of 1 lemon
salt and pepper

Heat the oil and fry the onion and garlic until soft. Add the lentils, cumin, coriander and water and bring to the boil. Lower the heat, cover and simmer for 40-50 minutes, until the lentils are soft but not mushy and the water is absorbed. Mix in the grated lemon rind and juice. Season to taste and leave to cool. Serve at room temperature.

Laban salateen
*Cucumber and yoghurt salad

Lebanon

Serves 4

Each serving: 81 kcal/339 kJ, 10 g carbohydrate, 1 g fibre, 7 g protein, 1 g fat

1 large cucumber, diced
a little salt
480 ml/17 fl oz low-fat plain yoghurt (see page 45)

2-3 cloves garlic, crushed
2 tbsp finely chopped fresh mint
pepper, to taste

Put the cucumber into a sieve and sprinkle lightly with salt. Leave to drain for 30 minutes, rinse off the salt and drain again.

Mix a few tablespoons of the yoghurt with the garlic, add the mixture to the rest of the yoghurt and mix well. Stir in the drained cucumber, mint and pepper.

Fattoush   *Syria*
**Bread salad   See photograph, page 100

Serves 4

Each serving: 113 kcal/475 kJ, 15 g carbohydrate, 4 g fibre, 4 g protein, 4 g fat

l large cucumber, diced
a little salt
1 bunch spring onions, cut into 5
cm/2 in slices
225 g/8 oz tomatoes, chopped
2 tbsp chopped fresh parsley
2 tbsp chopped fresh mint

1 tbsp chopped fresh coriander
(optional)
juice of 1 lemon
1 clove garlic, crushed
1 tbsp olive oil
pepper, to taste
1 wholemeal pitta bread

Put the cucumber into a sieve and sprinkle lightly with salt. Leave to drain for 30 minutes, rinse off the salt and drain again.

Mix all the ingredients except the pitta bread and chill.

When ready to serve, toast the pitta bread and break into small pieces. Mix into the salad and serve immediately while the pitta is still crisp.

Tabbouleh   *Lebanon*
*Cracked wheat salad

Serves 4

Each serving: 188 kcal/792 kJ, 35 g carbohydrate, 4 g fibre, 6 g protein, 5 g fat

150 g/5 oz burghul (see page 25),
soaked for 1 hour
1 small bunch spring onions or 1
Spanish onion, finely chopped
2 tomatoes, chopped
salt and pepper

50 g/2 oz fresh parsley, finely
chopped
25 g/1 oz fresh mint, finely
chopped
4 tbsp lemon juice
1 tbsp olive oil
vine leaves or lettuce, to serve

Drain the burghul and squeeze out with your hands. Spread out to dry for about half an hour on a clean teacloth.

Put the dried burghul into a bowl and mix in all the remaining ingredients. Serve on a dish, lined with vine leaves or lettuce.

Salatah ma'ah al-bourtokal   *Middle East*
**Orange and onion salad

Serves 4

Each serving: 111 kcal/465 kJ, 20 g carbohydrate, 4 g fibre, 2 g protein, 4 g fat

3 large oranges, peeled and thinly
sliced
1 Spanish onion, thinly sliced

6 black olives, stoned and halved
1 tbsp olive oil
3 tbsp orange juice

Arrange the orange and onion slices in layers and garnish with the olives. Mix together the oil and the orange juice and pour over the oranges.

Jitomates rellenos
**Stuffed tomato salad

Mexico

See photograph, page 100

Serves 4

Each serving: 78 kcal/327 kJ, 10 g carbohydrate, 4 g fibre, 4 g protein, 2 g fat

4 large tomatoes
4 lettuce leaves
25 g/1 oz courgettes, grated
25 g/1 oz carrots, grated
15 g/½ oz almonds, shelled and
    chopped
25 g/1 oz Spanish onion, grated
25 g/1 oz celery, grated

25 g/1 oz raisins
½ tsp dill seed
1 tbsp chopped fresh parsley
½ tsp dried thyme
150 ml/¼ pint smatana (see
    page 26) or Greek yoghurt
grated rind of ½ orange
1 canned red pimiento, thinly
    sliced

Stand the tomatoes on their stalk ends and make 5-6 cuts almost through to the bottom. Arrange them, stalk ends down, on the lettuce leaves. The tomatoes will then open, fan-like.

Mix together all the ingredients with the exception of the pimiento. Carefully spoon a little of the mixture into each cut. Alternatively, arrange it attractively beside the tomatoes. Garnish with curled strips of the pimiento. Chill until ready to serve.

Ensalada de topinambur
*Jerusalem artichoke salad

Mexico

Serves 4

Each serving: 20 kcal/86 kJ, 5 g carbohydrate, 1 g fibre, 2 g protein, negligible fat

450 g/1 lb Jerusalem artichokes,
    unpeeled and well scrubbed
salt

juice of 1 lime
2 tbsp chopped fresh parsley

Cook the artichokes in boiling salted water until tender but still firm. This will take 10-15 minutes but keep a careful watch, prodding the smallest ones first with the point of a knife. Remove the artichokes from the water as they are cooked.

Drain and slice the artichokes, and toss in the lime juice while still warm. Serve at room temperature, sprinkled with parsley.

Ensalada de papas con camarones
*Potato and prawn salad

Mexico

Serves 4 as a main dish, 6 as a starter

Each serving for 4: 174 kcal/729 kJ, 30 g carbohydrate, 3 g fibre, 12 g protein, 2 g fat
Each serving for 6: 116 kcal/486 kJ, 20 g carbohydrate, 2 g fibre, 8 g protein, 1 g fat

450 g/1 lb unpeeled potatoes
100 g/3½ oz cooked shelled
  prawns
1 stalk celery, finely chopped
4 spring onions, finely chopped

Dressing:
½ tsp dried tarragon
1 × 284 ml/9½ fl oz carton smatana
  (see page 26) or Greek yoghurt
1 tsp wine vinegar
1 clove garlic, crushed
1 tsp Dijon mustard
pepper, to taste

Boil the potatoes in their skins, peel, cut into large cubes and cool. Put them into a bowl with the prawns, celery and spring onions, reserving a few prawns and green onion tops for garnish.

Make the dressing: grind the tarragon to a powder with a pestle and mortar, or rub well between the fingers, and mix it with the smatana, wine vinegar, garlic, mustard and pepper. Stir the dressing lightly into the potatoes.

Serve garnished with the reserved prawns and onions.

Ensalada de verduras
**Mixed vegetable salad

Latin America

Serves 6

Each serving: 113 kcal/474 kJ, 15 g carbohydrate, 6 g fibre, 3 g protein, 5 g fat

225 g/8 oz cauliflower, divided into
  florets
225 g/8 oz carrots, cut lengthways
  if large
225 g/8 oz tiny new Jersey mid
  potatoes
225 g/8 oz tiny French beans, left
  whole

225 g/8 oz courgettes, sliced
225 g/8 oz small leeks, sliced
  lengthways

Dressing:
2 tbsp sunflower oil
2 tsp wine vinegar
½ tsp Dijon mustard
salt and pepper

Steam each vegetable individually until just cooked; a microwave is excellent for this. Cool the ingredients a little and when they are easy to handle, arrange on a very large platter. Make the dressing: stir all the ingredients together and then use to brush the vegetables very lightly while still warm. Serve at room temperature.

STAPLE
ACCOMPANIMENTS

In their traditional forms, meals in most countries incorporated rice, breads, grains and pasta, cooked with, or accompanied by, a protein and a vegetable dish. Poverty ensured that there were lavish helpings of the grain products and modest portions of the animal-derived proteins, which were often cooked in a liberal amount of fat. In this context, the fat was a small proportion of the meal. As people have become more affluent, and as these dishes have become absorbed into Western diets, the portions of protein dishes together with their fats have increased while the quantity of the grain accompaniments has decreased.

We should aim to return to the old way of eating, where small amounts of the protein food were accompanied by large quantities of the staple grains, supplemented with fresh vegetables.

RICE

White rice is the traditional staple in many countries in the East and Middle East as well as in Latin America. Basmati is used in India and Pakistan, a round rice in oriental cooking and Patna in Latin America. However, people with diabetes should eat only high-fibre whole rice on a regular basis, and the majority of recipes in this book have been adapted to use brown rice, with excellent results.

Plain boiled brown rice is a nutritious accompaniment to many of the dishes in this book. When served with dried bean dishes it enhances the protein in the pulses.

Brown rice has more flavour than white; some varieties are a little more chewy but the grains seldom stick together when cooking.

Suggested types of brown rice to accompany and include in dishes in this book are:

- Long-grain American or Australian, which have a light husk and are a good choice for people becoming used to brown rice
- Long-grain organic, which has a stronger husk, is a little more chewy but has a superior flavour
- Round Italian brown risotto rice for dishes containing stock: the grains swell and absorb the flavour.

Preparation

Brown rice, especially the coarser forms, can be very dusty. First pick it over and discard any bits of grit. Then put the rice into a bowl with plenty of water and agitate it with the hands. Allow the grains to sink to the bottom and pour off the cloudy water. Repeat until the water is clear. Drain.

Cooking

*Per portion: 178 kcal/750 kJ, 45 g carbohydrate, 2 g fibre, 3 g protein, 1 g fat

Allow 50 g/2 oz per person. Using a measuring jug, measure the rice into a saucepan with a well-fitting lid. Cover with twice the volume of cold water. Bring to the boil, cover and simmer for 30-40 minutes, according to the variety (until the water is absorbed). Test after 30 minutes, adding a little boiling water if necessary. Alternatively, cook according to the package directions.

Amarjit's jaul   *India*
*Spiced brown rice

Serves 4

Each serving: 228 kcal/958 kJ, 45 g carbohydrate, 3 g fibre, 5 g protein, 4 g fat

2 tsp sunflower oil
1 small onion, finely chopped
225 g/8 oz long-grain brown rice, washed and drained
½ green chilli, finely chopped

1 clove garlic
½ tsp garam masala
300 ml/½ pint stock, or ½ stock cube dissolved in 300 ml/½ pint water

Heat the oil in a non-stick saucepan and fry the onion until lightly browned. Add the rice, chilli, garlic and garam masala and stir, coating the grains of rice with the oil. Add the stock and bring to the boil. Cover and simmer, on as low a heat as possible, for 30-35 minutes, until the rice is cooked and the water is absorbed.

Punjabi jaul
*Punjabi salted rice

India

Serves 4

Each serving: 282 kcal/1186 kJ, 55 g carbohydrate, 5 g fibre, 7 g protein, 6 g fat

25 g/1 oz polyunsaturated
  margarine
1 small onion, very finely chopped
225 g/8 oz basmati rice, washed
  and drained

500 ml/17 fl oz water
1 tsp ground coriander
salt, to taste
3 bay leaves
200 g/7 oz shelled peas, fresh or
  frozen

Melt the margarine, add the onion and fry very gently until golden. Add the rice, water, coriander, salt and the bay leaves. Bring to the boil, cover and simmer for 7 minutes. Add the peas, bring back to the boil, cover and simmer for a further 7-8 minutes, or until the rice is cooked and the water absorbed.
  Serve with vegetable or meat curries or with tandoori dishes.

Baghala pilav
*Rice with broad beans

Middle East

Serves 4

Each serving: 216 kcal/907 kJ, 45 g carbohydrate, 4 g fibre, 7 g protein, 2 g fat

4 spring onions, or 1 small Spanish
  onion
1 tsp sunflower oil
½ tsp ground coriander
170 g/6 oz long-grain brown rice

600 ml/1 pint water
170 g/6 oz shelled broad beans
2 tbsp chopped fresh parsley

Fry the onions for a few minutes in the oil in a non-stick saucepan. Add the coriander, rice and the water and bring to the boil. Cover and simmer for 15 minutes. Add the beans and continue simmering for a further 15 minutes, or until the rice is cooked and the water absorbed. Stir in the parsley and serve hot or cold.

Masoor dhal
*Red lentil purée

India

Serves 4

Each serving: 110 kcal/460 kJ, 15 g carbohydrate, 4 g fibre, 7 g protein, 2 g fat

100 g/3½ oz red lentils, washed
300 ml/½ pint water
½ tsp turmeric
½ tsp ground cumin
½ tsp ground coriander

pinch of chilli powder
1 × 200 g/7 oz can tomatoes,
   drained and chopped
salt, to taste
1 tsp sunflower oil
1 large onion, thinly sliced

Put all the ingredients with the exception of the oil and the onion into a pan. Bring to the boil, cover and simmer gently for 1½ hours. Process in a food processor or beat until smooth, adding a little salt to taste. If the dhal is too liquid, reduce it by cooking it over a medium heat for a few minutes, stirring all the time.

· Heat the oil in a non-stick pan and fry the onion, covered, until beginning to brown. Serve the dhal in a preheated bowl, garnished with the onion.

GRAINS

Burghul pilav
*Cracked wheat

Middle East

Serves 4

Each serving: 236 kcal/992 kJ, 45 g carbohydrate, 2 g fibre, 7 g protein, 4 g fat

15 g/½ oz polyunsaturated
   margarine
1 small onion, finely chopped
250 g/9 oz small grain burghul (see
   page 26), washed and drained

150 ml/¼ pint boiling water
salt and pepper

Melt the margarine in a non-stick frying pan and fry the onion until brown. Add the burghul and fry gently, turning the wheat in the margarine with a wooden fork until the grains are coated. Add the boiling water, a little at a time, and heat the grains through. Season, turn off the heat, cover the pan and set aside for 10 minutes.

Note: In this unconventional recipe the burghul is not cooked, merely heated through. Any of the herbs, spices, fruits or vegetables that are added to rice pilavs may be used with this basic recipe.

Chapati
Unleavened flat breads

India

See photograph, page 117

Makes 12

Each chapati: 66 kcal/278 kJ, 15 g carbohydrate, 2 g fibre, 3 g protein, negligible fat

225 g/8 oz ata flour (see page 25)
  or finely ground wholemeal
  flour

pinch of salt
about 200 ml/7 fl oz water

Sift the flour and salt into a bowl. Mix in enough water to make a medium-soft dough and knead well for 5 minutes. Cover and set aside for 30 minutes.

Divide the dough into 12 equal sized balls. On a lightly floured surface, roll each ball into a 15 cm/6 in circle. (They can be frozen at this stage if interleaved with plastic).

Heat a heavy-based ungreased iron griddle, frying pan or *tawa*, a convex chapati pan, take the first chapati and cook until it begins to bubble. Turn it over and cook the other side. As the second side cooks, press the top firmly here and there with a pad made of folded kitchen paper. This makes the chapatis puff up.

As they are cooked, stack the chapatis, covering them with a towel to keep them soft and warm. Serve with curries.

Saag paratha
Spinach paratha

India

See photograph, page 117

Makes 8

Each paratha: 130 kcal/545 kJ, 20 g carbohydrate, 4 g fibre, 4 g protein, 5 g fat

225 g/8 oz wholemeal flour
100 g/3½ oz cooked spinach, well
  drained, chopped and cooled

40 g/1½ oz polyunsaturated mar-
  garine
7 tbsp water

Mix the flour with the spinach and 15 g/½ oz margarine. Mix with enough water to make a soft dough. Knead well and set aside to rest until ready to cook.

Divide the dough into eight even-size pieces and form into balls. Roll each ball into a 15 cm/6 in circle.

Heat a heavy-based ungreased frying pan or Indian *tawa* and cook the paratha for 2-3 minutes on each side over a low heat. When they are all cooked, grease each with the minimum amount of margarine on each side and fry gently until they are lightly browned. Serve hot with curries or tandoori dishes.

Naan
*Yeast-raised flatbread

India

Makes 4

Each naan: 234 kcal/983 kJ, 40 g carbohydrate, 6 g fibre, 10 g protein, 5 g fat

*225 g/8 oz soft fine wholemeal
  flour*
¼ tsp salt
15 g/½ oz fresh yeast

1 tbsp sunflower oil
*150 ml/¼ pint low-fat plain yoghurt
  (see page 45)*

Sift the flour into a warmed bowl with the salt. Rub in the yeast, add the oil and the yoghurt. Knead well on a lightly floured work surface until smooth. Cover the dough and leave in a warm place until doubled in size.

Punch the dough down and divide it into four balls. Roll each ball into a large pear shape about 5 mm/¼ in thick. Put them on to a floured surface and cover. Leave in a warm place for about 30 minutes, until they are beginning to rise again.

Set the grill at maximum heat, grease the grill rack lightly and grill the naan as near as possible to the source of the heat without burning. When one side is brown, turn and grill the other side. The naan should puff up well but flatten again as they cool.

Serve immediately, spread with a skimming of polyunsaturated margarine and sprinkled with sesame or white poppy seeds if required. Serve with tandoori dishes, kebabs or curries.

Saag paratha (*top*, see page 115); Naan (*centre left*); Chapati (*below*, see page 115).
OVERLEAF: A selection of fruits: pears, bananas, grapes, apples, yellow and brown dates; papaya (prepared – *left*, see page 125); mango (prepared – *top centre*, see page 124); rambutan (*centre foreground*, see page 124); passion fruit (*centre right*, see page 125); lychees (*in bowl*, see page 124).

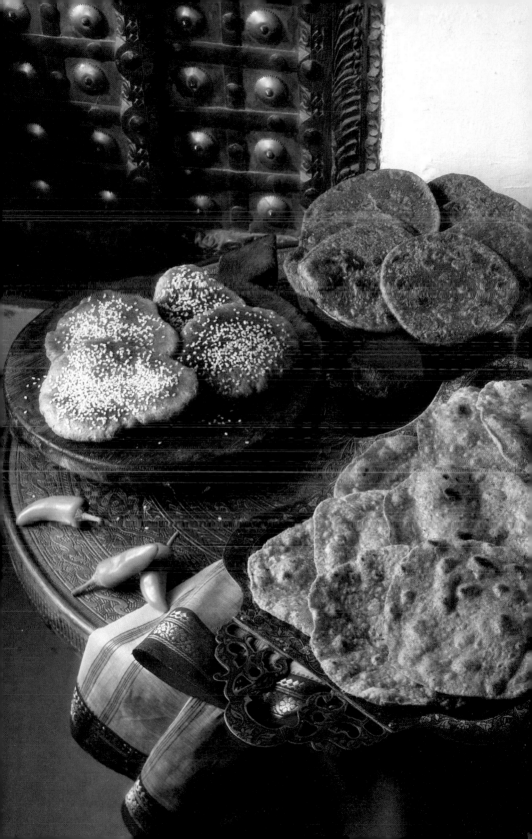

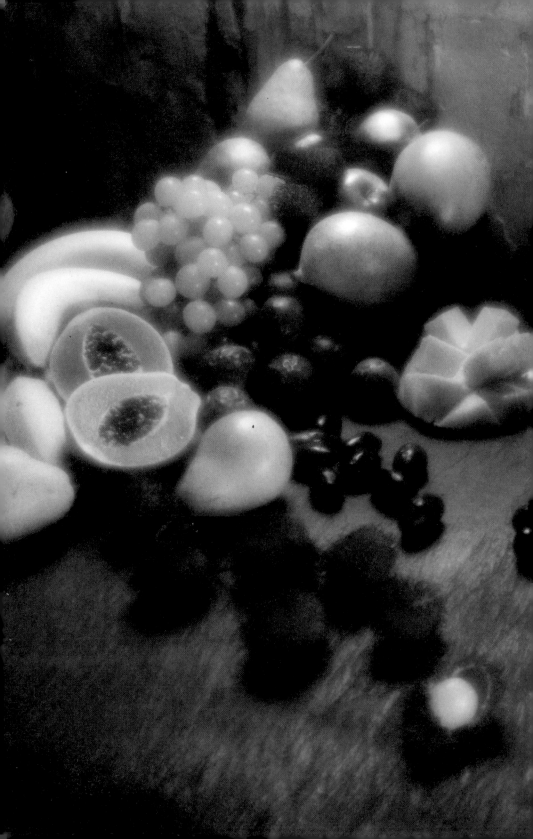

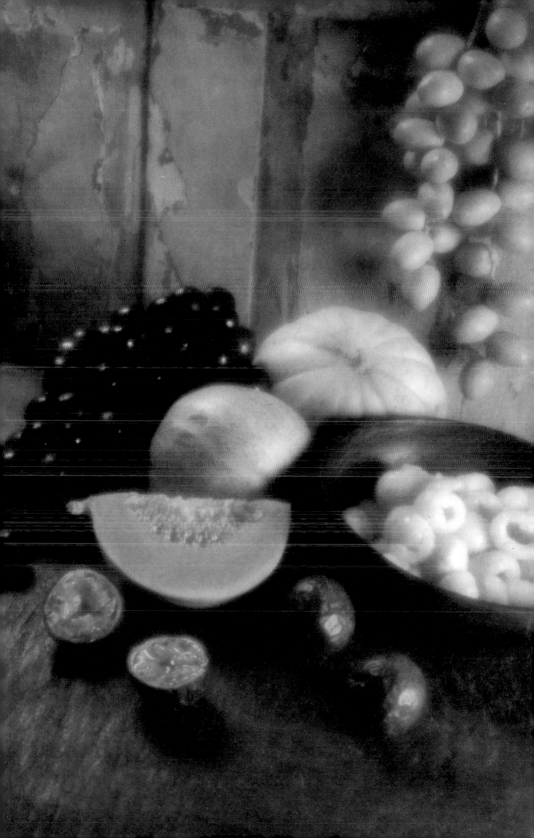

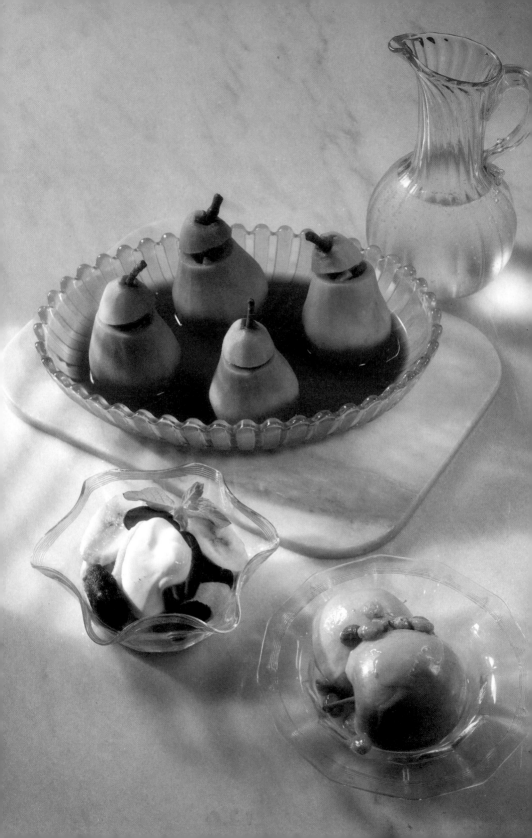

PUDDINGS

Many exotic and unusual fruits are now available from the larger supermarkets, some looking seductive and appealing, others with coarse, wrinkled or blemished skins which belie the wonderful aromas, textures and flavours that are revealed once you have solved the mysteries of their preparation. I have listed the countries from which each originated. Most are now grown much more widely as they are in great demand throughout the world.

There is, of course, natural sugar in all fruit, but it is very low in comparison with puddings and cakes containing added sugar. In fruit, the sugar is combined with fibre which helps to release it slowly into the bloodstream.

In some recipes in this book, dried and fresh fruits appear in starters and main dishes, as they are served in their countries of origin (for example, the courgettes stuffed with dates and nuts, see page 43). From the point of view of re-educating tastes to the new way of nutrition, this can be helpful. Puddings have been fixed in the minds of most of us from childhood as treats at the end of a meal. By eating sweet foods at different stages of a meal, they are taken out of their star role and included in a more natural way, while satisfying a desire for something a little sweet.

All the fruits described in this section are simple to prepare, look beautiful when presented in pretty dishes, and will fit happily into menus made up from the recipes in this book.

One or two of the recipes call for unsweetened fruit juices, such as apricot and orange (see page 123). These exotic combinations are now available in many of the large supermarkets and make excellent sweetening agents in sugar-free recipes.

*Tropical fruit salad   Far East

Serves 6

Each serving: 90 kcal/376 kJ, 20 g carbohydrate, 3 g fibre, 2 g protein, negligible fat

250 ml/8 fl oz unsweetened orange and passion fruit juice
1 small melon, skinned, seeded and cubed
1 papaya, skinned, seeded and cubed

1 mango, skinned, stone removed and cubed
2 passion fruit, flesh scooped out, seeds reserved
2 bananas

Agasim memoula'im (*top, see page 123); Balatt wa-moze (*centre left*, see page 123); Toufah bil-mishmish (*below*, see page 122).

Put the fruit juice into a glass bowl. Add the melon, papaya, mango and passion fruit with the peeled and sliced bananas. Arrange the passion fruit seeds decoratively over the fruit salad. Serve chilled or at room temperature.

Note: For choice and preparation of the fruits, see individual fruits, pages 124–5.

Khoshaf   *Iran*
**Dried fruit salad

Serves 8

Each serving: 132 kcal/553 kJ, 20 g carbohydrate, 9 g fibre, 3 g protein, 5 g fat

225 g/8 oz dried apricots
50 g/2 oz dried prunes
50 g/2 oz seedless raisins or sultanas
50 g/2 oz almonds, blanched and halved

25 g/1 oz pistachio nuts or pine kernels
2 tbsp orange flower water, or 1 tbsp rose water

Put the fruit into a large bowl with all the other ingredients. Add enough water to cover. Cover the bowl and refrigerate for 2 days or up to a week. Serve on its own or with yoghurt.

Toufah bil-mishmish   *Middle East*
*Apples in apricot and orange nectar   See photograph,
Serves 4   page 120

Each serving: 126 kcal/530 kJ, 25 g carbohydrate, 2 g fibre, 1 g protein, 3 g fat

350 ml/12 fl oz unsweetened apricot and orange nectar or unsweetened orange juice
25 g/1 oz sultanas

15 g/½ oz polyunsaturated margarine
4 Granny Smiths or other hard dessert apples
1 tbsp cornflour

Put the fruit juice into a saucepan with the sultanas and the margarine. Bring to the boil. Halve, peel and core the apples and put them into the juice. Simmer gently for 7-10 minutes, or until soft but still whole.

Mix the cornflour with a little cold water. Remove the apples to a serving dish, cut side down. Stir the cornflour mixture into the juice and simmer for 2-3 minutes. Pour over the apples and chill.

Balatt wa-moze
Middle East

*Banana and date dessert   See photograph, page 120

Serves 4

Each serving: 122 kcal/511 kJ, 25 g carbohydrate, 1 g fibre, 4 g protein, 1 g fat

150 g/5 oz fresh dates or 100 g/
   3½ oz dried dates
2 bananas, peeled and sliced

250 ml/8 fl oz low-fat plain yoghurt
   (see page 45)

Prepare the fresh dates by cutting off the stalk end and popping the date out. Discard the stones and skins and cut the flesh into half. Dried dates do not need skinning; simply quarter them and remove the stones if they have any.

Arrange a layer of bananas in a small serving dish. Cover with the dates and top with a layer of bananas. Pour over the yoghurt, cover the dish and refrigerate for several hours or overnight to allow the yoghurt to absorb the flavour of the dates.

Agasim memoula'im
Israel

*Stuffed pears   See photograph, page 120

Serves 4

Each serving: 101 kcal/426 kJ, 15 g carbohydrate, 3 g fibre, 1 g protein, 2 g fat

Stuffing:
25 g/1 oz sultanas
15 g/½ oz shelled walnuts,
   chopped
½ tsp ground cinnamon

150 ml/¼ pint red wine
2 tbsp concentrated unsweetened
   apple juice
1 strip lemon rind
100 ml/3 fl oz water
1 small stick cinnamon
3 cloves
4 ripe pears

Mix together the sultanas, walnuts and ground cinnamon. Put the wine, apple juice, lemon rind, water, cinnamon stick and cloves into a small saucepan and bring to the boil.

Heat the oven to 180°C/350°F/Gas 4. Cut 2.5 cm/1 in from the stem end of the pears and set aside. Using a small teaspoon, scoop out the cores and sufficient flesh to leave room for the stuffing. Peel the pears and stuff them. Replace the stem ends and arrange the pears in an ovenproof dish just large enough to accommodate them. It may be necessary to cut a little off the base of each pear to enable it to stand upright.

Pour the wine mixture over the pears, cover and bake for 45-60 minutes or until the pears are cooked.

Place the pears on a serving dish. Pour the cooking liquid back into the saucepan and reduce to a thick syrup. Pour over the pears and chill before serving.

*Lychees   *China*

A lychee is a small, unprepossessing looking fruit, the size of a small plum with a thin, rough, dark brown skin. Peel it off and you will reveal a pearly white flesh with a distinctively perfumed aroma. Serve them after a Chinese meal.

Each fruit: 6 kcal/27 kJ, 2 g carbohydrate, negligible fibre, negligible protein, negligible fat

Choice: select even-size lychees. Reject any which feel comparatively light. They may have dried out.

Preparation: using a sharp pointed knife, peel back the skin and remove the stone.

Serve: whole on their own, in fruit salads or in sweet-sour dishes.

*Rambutan   *Indonesia and Thailand*

A rambutan is very similar to a lychee but its shell is covered with soft spines.

Each fruit: 6 kcal/27 kJ, 2 g carbohydrate, negligible fibre, negligible protein, negligible fat

Choose, prepare and serve: exactly as for lychees (see above). In Thailand cooks cut and peel the shells back to resemble delicate flowers.

*Mango   *Brazil and India*

A mango is a large, heavy fruit resembling in shape a giant plum. It may be green, gold, red or orange. Its flesh is a bright dark yellow with the most wonderful flavour and aroma.

Each fruit: 133 kcal/557 kJ, 35 g carbohydrate, 3 g fibre, 1 g protein, negligible fat

Choice: a ripe mango yields to medium pressure.

Preparation: mangos have a large stone which clings to the flesh and makes it a little tricky to remove. Lay the fruit on a board with the narrow side facing you. Cut through the mango vertically 1 cm/½ in from the centre with a large stainless steel knife. Make a similar cut 1 cm/½ in from the other side of the centre. You will be left with two side sections and a central section containing the stone.

   Make parallel cuts on one section at 1 cm/½ in intervals through the flesh almost to the skin. Make similar cuts across the fruit, making squares. Do the same with the second section.

Serve: turn the sections inside out and serve. Alternatively, for speed, serve the sections with spoons for scooping out at table. They may also be peeled and cubed and used in fruit salads.

Persimmon or Sharon fruit: Israel

This fruit looks like a large yellowish tomato with a large green leafy stalk.

Each fruit: 129 kcal/542 kJ, 35 g carbohydrate, fibre n/a, 1 g protein, 1 g fat

Choice: choose fruit which are soft to the touch.

Preparation: wash and dry.

Serve: cut the fruit in halves and serve with teaspoons. The skin may be eaten.

*Passion fruit *Brazil and Israel*

Do not be put off by the appearance of these fruits which gives the impression that they have passed their sell-by date. These plum-size fruit have a hard purple-brown wizened-looking skin, but a delightfully refreshing flavour.

Each fruit: 6 kcal/24 kJ, 1 g carbohydrate, 3 g fibre, 1 g protein, negligible fat

Choice: passion fruit are ripe when the skin looks dimpled.

Preparation: cut in half and scoop out the fruit and seeds with a teaspoon.

Serve: pile whole fruits on to a serving dish and decorate with flowers or leaves. Give guests a small spoon and a fruit knife so they may cut the fruit at table and scoop out the fragrant liquid. Alternatively, use the flesh and seeds to decorate fruit salads and other desserts.

*Papaya *Brazil and Mexico*

This fruit looks a little like a large, irregular, smooth-skinned, yellowish-green pear. It has a pinky-orange flesh which tastes a little like melon.

Each fruit: 101 kcal/425 kJ, 25 g carbohydrate, 1 g fibre, 1 g protein, negligible fat

Choice: buy when the skin begins to turn yellow and it yields a little to light pressure at the stalk end.

Preparation: cut in half lengthways and scoop out the seeds or peel and slice.

Serve: place the halves on individual dishes sprinkled with lime juice. They are eaten with a small spoon. Alternatively, the peeled fruit can be sliced or chopped and arranged attractively on a plate or added to fruit salads.

INDEX

Page numbers in *italic* refer to the illustrations